Vanessa,

I hope you get a
lot of this !!

# Praise for Doctor Thurston's Other Works

## Death of Compassion

"An engrossing portrait of medicine today and an impassioned cry of concern for medicine tomorrow, this is a very worthwhile book."

**—Rabbi Harold Kushner,**
author of *When Bad Things Happen to Good People.*

"Thurston's real life examples of the dire consequences of basing medical decisions solely on economic expediency are chilling."

**—Library Journal**

"Often with satirical wit, sometimes with heartrending depictions of utter anguish, Thurston's stories unfold with the same fascination as an intriguing novel."

**—Doctor Michael DeBakey,**
**Chancellor Baylor College of Medicine**

## 1000 Questions About Your Pregnancy

"Dr. Thurston has asked and answered a thousand questions about pregnancy in a book that is easy to read, comprehensive, and scientifically founded; patients as well as physicians can benefit from his sound advice."

**—Susan B. Cox, MD, FACOG,**
**Associate Professor of Obstetrics and Gynecology,**
**University of Texas Southwestern Medical School**

"I had the pleasure of knowing Dr. Thurston during his years as a medical student at Baylor College of Medicine. Without a doubt, he was one of the finest and brightest students with whom I have had contact during my many years of teaching medical students. He is currently a superb, knowledgeable clinician."

**—Raymond H. Kaufamn, MD, FACOG,**
**Chairman Emeritus, Department of Obstetrics and**
**Gynecology, Baylor College of Medicine**

# DISROBE *completely*

# DISROBE
## Completely

Real Life Cases REVEAL
the State of American Medicine.

## JEFFREY M. THURSTON, MD, FACOG

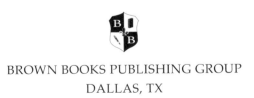

BROWN BOOKS PUBLISHING GROUP
DALLAS, TX

# DISROBE COMPLETELY

## Real Life Cases REVEAL the State of American Medicine.

Manufactured in the United States.

For information, please contact:

Brown Books Publishing Group

16200 North Dallas Parkway, Suite 170

Dallas, Texas 75248

www.brownbooks.com

972-381-0009

A New Era in Publishing™

ISBN-13: 978-1-933285-69-6

ISBN-10: 1-933285-69-6

LCCN: 2006938544

1 2 3 4 5 6 7 8 9 10

To Allison, Andy, Kelly, and Ashley:

Their love, gentleness, and kindness

are evident to all.

# Contents

To the Reader                                                    xi
Preface                                                          xiii
Foreword                                                         xvii
Acknowledgements                                                 xix
Introduction                                                     xxi

## Part 1

### Disrobe Completely: Naiveté                                 1

Boldly in Red . . . . . . . . . . . . . . . . . . . . . . . . . . . . . . . . . . . . . . 2
Hither and Yonder . . . . . . . . . . . . . . . . . . . . . . . . . . . . . . . . 5
Weight by History . . . . . . . . . . . . . . . . . . . . . . . . . . . . . . . . 8
Toe Tag . . . . . . . . . . . . . . . . . . . . . . . . . . . . . . . . . . . . . . . . .12
Aequanimitas . . . . . . . . . . . . . . . . . . . . . . . . . . . . . . . . . . . .18
The Strong Survive . . . . . . . . . . . . . . . . . . . . . . . . . . . . . . . 22
My Tool . . . . . . . . . . . . . . . . . . . . . . . . . . . . . . . . . . . . . . . . 29
Spanish Inquisition . . . . . . . . . . . . . . . . . . . . . . . . . . . . . . . 33

## Part 2

### Put the Gown on So It Opens in Front: Experience  41

Not in Kansas Anymore . . . . . . . . . . . . . . . . . . . . . . . . . . 42
A Radical Concept . . . . . . . . . . . . . . . . . . . . . . . . . . . . . . . 53
Good Grief . . . . . . . . . . . . . . . . . . . . . . . . . . . . . . . . . . . . . 58
Let 'Em See You Sweat . . . . . . . . . . . . . . . . . . . . . . . . . . . 65
Big Sucker, Idn'it? . . . . . . . . . . . . . . . . . . . . . . . . . . . . . . . .74

Not a Nice Word . . . . . . . . . . . . . . . . . . . . . . . . . . . . . . . . . . . . . 82

The Bad Disease . . . . . . . . . . . . . . . . . . . . . . . . . . . . . . . . . . . . . . 87

A Little Bit in Love . . . . . . . . . . . . . . . . . . . . . . . . . . . . . . . . . . . 99

Sacred Trust . . . . . . . . . . . . . . . . . . . . . . . . . . . . . . . . . . . . . . . . .108

Shell Shocked. . . . . . . . . . . . . . . . . . . . . . . . . . . . . . . . . . . . . . . .123

This Is Embarrassing, But. . . . . . . . . . . . . . . . . . . . . . . . . . . . . . .129

# Part 3

## Have a Seat on the Table: Reality                    135

Patient Name and Group Number . . . . . . . . . . . . . . . . . . . . . . .137

Noneconomic Damages . . . . . . . . . . . . . . . . . . . . . . . . . . . . . . .154

Something Bad Wrong . . . . . . . . . . . . . . . . . . . . . . . . . . . . . . . .166

Teaching? . . . . . . . . . . . . . . . . . . . . . . . . . . . . . . . . . . . . . . . . . .183

# Part 4

## Scoot All the Way to the Edge: Approaches       187

The Problem. . . . . . . . . . . . . . . . . . . . . . . . . . . . . . . . . . . . . . . . .188

The Solution: Managed Competition?. . . . . . . . . . . . . . . . . . . . 205

Some Answers. . . . . . . . . . . . . . . . . . . . . . . . . . . . . . . . . . . . . 213

Conclusion. . . . . . . . . . . . . . . . . . . . . . . . . . . . . . . . . . . . . . . . 230

## Notes                                             237

# To the Reader

This is a work of nonfiction. The stories of individual patients are true, and the people are real. My patients' names have been changed in the interest of protecting their privacy. Where relevant, the names of institutions and prominent public figures have been left unchanged.

While I have reconstructed the events to the best of my recollection, the dialogue is, in some places, an approximation. Nevertheless, the lessons learned from each patient and each encounter are true.

Finally, the opinions about how to deal with the crisis in our health care system are strictly my own. They may not represent the positions of any of my colleagues or of the institutions with which I am, or have been, involved.

—JMT

# Preface

It has been ten years since the release of the first edition of this book. That first edition was titled *Death of Compassion*. As I witnessed the changing landscape of American health care, I felt a tremendous need to warn and inform the public of the very real dangers on the horizon pertaining to the quality of medical care that they might soon find available. *Disrobe Completely* is an effort to help people understand that the doctor-patient relationship is the essence of what makes our system the envy of the world. The only way for people to truly understand that relationship is to achieve some understanding of who doctors really are, what makes them tick, and how they got to be that way. Once the public acknowledges the centrality of the relationship with their personal physician, they can begin to defend that relationship when it comes under assault.

It would be wonderful if I could say there have been tremendous changes for the better in America's health care system since 1995, but that, unfortunately, would not ring true. There are new stories in *Disrobe Completely*, but you will find all of the stories, new and old, from the education, training, and practice of a physician in the latter half of the twentieth century just as humorous, informative, heartwarming, and relevant as they were when first written. But that doesn't change the fact that America's health care system is in a shambles!

In 1995, we were facing not only the prospect of managed care radically changing the third-party payment system but also HMOs wresting control of decision making from physicians and patients. The backlash of that tendency was felt in the boardrooms of every insurance company in America, and managed care companies gradually learned to quiet their vocal emphasis on cost containment and change the names of their HMOs to such monikers as "managed choice," and "direct access." Never mind that most of the changes were superficial at best. Patients had become furious with the inability of their physicians to make medical choices and with their own inability to choose those physicians. Plaintiff's attorneys sensed an opening, and huge corporations had multimillion dollar judgments against them as courts decided that they were indeed responsible for the life-altering sacrifices they had demanded of their clients on the altar of improved profitability.

Today, we find a society with forty-five million people unable to access much of our system due to the lack of any type of insurance. While the most intrusive of the HMOs have been somewhat restrained in their ability to make health care decisions for which they are woefully ill-prepared, even insured patients continue to have either gross restrictions of or outrageously complicated systems of access and payment for outpatient, pharmaceutical, and inpatient care. Corporations that once offered full health care coverage can no longer afford to do so. Many switch each year to the most economical plan they can find, and even at that, their employees are now forced to pay a portion of the premiums. Smaller companies and self-employed business people often find it hard to obtain insurance at all unless at outrageous premiums that they simply cannot afford.

Many other companies have simply stopped offering health plans altogether. Giant corporations like General Motors and Ford face bankruptcy largely secondary to skyrocketing health care costs, the majority of which are generated not even by their producing employees but by the ever-expanding number of pensioned retirees.

Congress has made some changes. The Health Insurance Portability and Accountability Act of 1996 (PL 104 - 191 or HIPAA) was an attempt to improve patients' ability to change employers yet avoid riders for unreasonable periods on the coverages they needed the most. Instead, HIPAA was created—another behemoth federal bureaucracy whose intent was privacy and supposedly portability, but whose result was yet another layer of obfuscation and interference between the health care provider and patient. Each year, hundreds of thousands of patients are still forced to change doctors and hospitals because their employer has sought out yet another slightly more cost-effective benefits plan, which unfortunately includes a different list of "providers."

As the first wave of baby boomers—those born shortly after World War II—approaches age sixty-five, the nation faces the potential for a crisis of unprecedented proportions. Dire predictions of when both Medicare and Social Security will go broke are as common and varied as the experts who make them. But all the predictions have a common thread, and the future "don't look so hot," as we'd say in Texas. The federal government made a recent attempt to alleviate the plight of seniors as health care costs continue to skyrocket by instituting a prescription drug plan for Medicare. At this writing, the chances of obtaining even a modicum of understanding about the plan's functioning are "iffy" at best. In short, despite well-meaning legislators, the implementation has been a nightmare. On top of all this, physicians are so poorly compensated by Medicare (in many cases actually losing money for every visit) that in the very near future less than 20% of physicians may even accept Medicare patients into their practices. Not a good scenario as the number of patients over sixty-five mushrooms like a nuclear cloud.

One thing is certain. Patients will continue to want a relationship with a physician they can call their own, one who knows them and their family and has the capacity to form a relationship that actually allows the patient to be "cared for." As new federal elections approach, you can be sure that health-care delivery will once again be hotly debated, though perhaps overshadowed by Iraq, Iran, North Korea, and the Middle East. All I can do is encourage every one of you to fight for any chance at having a relationship with a physician who knows you and the right to choose who that is and in what facility you wish to receive care.

That means supporting some variant of consumer-driven health plans (CDHP), which include variants of the fledgling health savings accounts I advocated over ten years ago. The cost of health care must once again be directly related to the consumer, or market forces cannot correct rising costs and rising profits for those who feed off of the vulnerable. We should look at any method for handling our health costs that promotes personal responsibility. This would include employer-sponsored wellness initiatives from education about weight loss and exercise, smoking cessation, safer sex, nutritional education, and so on.

This means pushing your representatives for *national tort reform* in order to lower everyone's health care costs and boost all aspects of the nation's productivity and ability to compete.

This means innovative thinking when it comes to funding Social Security, Medicare, and helping the uninsured. It means vigorously supporting the politicians you feel have the best ideas. While I do not advocate it currently, it might eventually mean some sort of nationalized health care. Even if that happens, pay attention and fight for the legislators who recognize that your right to choose is fundamental to good care.

Just realize that you are getting older too, and where you may once have thought this wasn't really your problem, it is about to become everyone's problem in a very real way.

**Jeff Thurston, MD, FACOG**
Dallas 2007

# Foreword to
# Death of Compassion

by Dr. Michael DeBakey

Something is happening in American health care. It's been happening for some time now—right before our eyes. As national attention is focused on containing spiraling health care costs, the hidden price of that containment eats away at the heart of our medical-delivery system. The price of containment may be the doctor-patient relationship unless the danger of its erosion is recognized and certain misguided attempts at reform are redirected.

In more than fifty years of surgical practice, I have been dismayed at the recent escalating, tragic conflict between medical and financial priorities. As President of Baylor College of Medicine and Chairman of the Department of Surgery, and now as the college's chancellor, I have supervised the training of thousands of physicians. The disparate goals of physicians who were trained to put the patient's welfare first and those of the profit-driven, insurance-owned medical corporations are rapidly disillusioning physicians and patients alike. Increasingly, the sanctity of life is being subordinated to Mammon, and medical decisions are being dictated by those unqualified to do so. The patient's choices are being wrested, and the physician's authority is being expropriated—to the detriment of all.

If, in 1956, we had had the same commercial environment that we have today, we might never have developed the heart-lung machine that launched open-heart surgery, or synthetic aortic grafts, or mechanical assist devices for the failing heart, or any of a myriad of medical miracles that derived from the research of the academic medical centers of excellence. Today, our teaching institutions are threatened financially by the changing third-party payment system and the evaporation of research funds. In that environment, where will we find the answers to currently incurable diseases?

Dr. Thurston explores these issues with actual patient histories, firsthand accounts of the frustrations, and the dangers involved in profit-motivated, corporate medicine. Often with satirical wit, sometimes with heartrending depictions of utter anguish, his stories unfold with the same fascination as an intriguing novel.

While recognizing a need for some reform in our health system, Dr. Thurston opens our eyes to the dangers of "reforms" based solely on cost containment. Managed care may be here, but as it develops, we need to make certain that the interests of the patient remain paramount rather than being relegated to an obscure footnote.

As the self-appointed, health-policy "experts" continue to bombard the public with their ill-conceived but superficially seductive "health reforms," it is imperative that the public be alerted to the dire consequences of the nation's health and economy that will ensue. So turn the page and get an insider's view of a physician's world in 1995. Experience a glimpse of his training and of the cases that have shaped him as a person and a physician. But most of all take heed, because something disquieting is happening in the world of medicine. And when you experience its effects, you may not like it.

**Michael E. DeBakey, MD**
Chancellor and Distinguished Service Professor of Surgery
Director, DeBakey Heart Center
Baylor College of Medicine
Houston, Texas 1996

# Acknowledgements

I owe a tremendous debt of gratitude to my new publisher, Milli Brown. Without her faith in me and her vision for the potential in this book, the project would never have occurred at all. The entire crew at Brown Books has been fun, relaxed, upbeat, and a joy with which to work!

I am especially beholdin', as we say in Texas, to several individuals. Kathryn Grant, my editor, had the toughest job of all. Taking authors' words, which they really view more as their children, and then gently correcting the aspects and verbiage, which they at times had absurdly wrong, is truly a herculean task. Kathryn handled my fits of pique with panache, and unfailingly led me consistently in the "write" direction, and for that I am particularly grateful.

Ted Ruybal used his creative genius on the "look" of the book both inside and out. His covers were excellent and provocative, his use of space creative and his choice of fonts and layout pleasing to the reader's eye. Cindy Birne and Neal Kimmel worked tirelessly to find the improbable and then to arrange the impossible from endorsements and publicity angles to speaking engagements and book signings. With a message that I very much wanted to bring to public awareness, Cindy and Neal have been indispensable. My thanks as well to Rafael "the money man" Parra at Brown Books who looked after the numbers for all of us!

My thanks also, to my friend and first editor on *Death of Compassion*, now released . . . incredibly over a decade ago! Chris Tucker's support and organizational skills went a long way toward making a writer out of what was, at the time, simply a doctor with something he wanted to say.

I want also to thank Rice University and Baylor College of Medicine in Houston and the University of California Medical School in San Francisco for their outstanding programs that allowed me to enter the field of my choice with a solid academic and clinical background.

My partners at Walnut Hill Ob/Gyn in Dallas, doctors Jim Richards, John Bertrand, Jane Nokeberg, Julie Hagood, David Bookout, and my former partners

# Disrobe Completely

Henry Estess and Bernadine Bank all deserve my gratitude. Their patience, stories, constant support, and reliable call coverage have all contributed to this work.

Evelyn Scott, RN, my "rock," is my nurse of eighteen years and counting. She keeps me on time, in good humor, somewhat aware of what I am doing at all times, and without her, I would have failed on all fronts years ago.

My wife, Pat, deserves my gratitude for supporting this, the most recent of many endeavors beyond my usual seventy-hour work week. She encourages me to move forward with new projects as well as dusting off old ones that have rested for too long in the files or on the shelves of my library. There is no retirement, honey, just more and more life!

Thank you to my children—Allison, Andy, Ashley, and Kelly. Their unconditional love has buoyed me through each storm in recent years and will be a source of strength and comfort for me until my dying day.

I cannot forget my parents, Bob and Phyllis Thurston, without whose consistent love, support, and teaching I would not be who I am. I also owe a debt of gratitude to my big brother, Dr. Scott Thurston. In our childhood, he bested me in every contest, physical and mental, as older brothers are prone to do. It was that sibling rivalry in brotherly love that helped me to develop the willpower necessary for achieving my goals.

It often goes without saying, but it needs to be said more frequently and more forcefully, that anything I accomplish is really only possible through the power of the Holy Spirit and the use of the talents given to me by the Creator. May the constant support and guidance afforded me by God Almighty in the person of his son, Jesus Christ, my personal Lord and Savior, be passed on to others by my obedience and testimony.

Lastly, I wish to thank all of those women out there who answer the question, "Who's your doctor?" by giving my name. It is not only for your benefit that I write this book but also because of you that I feel so strongly. For the physician, his patients are his strength, his inspiration, his reason for being. They are, in fact, who he is.

—JMT

# Introduction

## I Used to be a Doctor

I used to be a doctor. You know, a physician. Someone who had patients that he cared for, looked after. Someone to whom people came for help because they didn't feel good, or they were scared or confused or injured.

No longer. Now they tell me I'm a health care provider. I no longer have patients, because people like you, who used to be patients, have become customers. You know, like, "I'm sorry, lady, you can't return the blouse just because you look lousy in it. Now move along, please, we've got lots of folks in line."

I'm a fifty-year-old obstetrician-gynecologist at a major private institution in Dallas, Texas. I came to this startling sense of enlightenment over ten years ago in late 1993 at one of the new breed of seminars, this one dealing with managed care and presented by a short, balding, gray-headed man with a goatee.

Mr. Goatee represented one of the huge, omnipotent companies in the health-insurance industry, the name of which you would no doubt recognize. Over the course of an hour and a half, he proceeded to lecture two hundred physicians on the inevitable changes to be wrought by impending health-care reform. These changes, he declared in a condescending tone, were to be imposed upon us from the outside, and we would finally have to conduct our business like every other organized human activity, with higher regard for purchaser satisfaction.

# Disrobe Completely

It was roughly three o'clock in the morning several weeks after the seminar when I was baptized into my new identity as health care provider. That may seem like an unusual time for the creative spirit to move me, but I do most of my writing while on call at the hospital. New babies don't always schedule their arrivals between the hours of nine and five, and that means plenty of waiting. Time to think.

That night, as I waited for Mother Nature once again, I was thinking about what Mr. Goatee had said. It occurred to me then, as I'm sure it did to others, that he hadn't the slightest idea what he was talking about. He may know his own business, but he had no idea what a physician is, what he does or believes, or what might be involved in becoming one.

And this gentleman was supposed to be an expert on health care reform. He represented the insurance industry, which is far more influential than the federal government in driving reform.

No doubt Mr. Goatee and his corporate cohorts would have their own definition of managed care and its sibling, managed competition. To me, these are umbrella terms for a widespread health care delivery system in which decisions about diagnosis and treatment are no longer made solely in the best interest of the patient by those most capable of making those decisions. Instead, the decisions are made by persons whose goal is the profitability of the payor. Patients are just now starting to realize that while their company's new health plan looked good initially with that $10 co-pay, they have very limited options as to where and from whom they can seek their health care.

Most of the doctors at that seminar knew that the practice of medicine differs markedly from the selling of small appliances or used cars. But what about our patients? (I mean, customers.) As I thought back on what Mr. Goatee had said, I wondered how many Americans he spoke for with his demands that we physicians must practice medicine by focusing on purchaser (i.e., insurer) satisfaction and conduct our business like every other organized human activity.

# Introduction

I don't know the answer to that question. The opinion polls tell us many things, but they don't tell us that. But I do know this: if Mr. Goatee's views are held by any significant portion of the American public, then a vast gulf has opened up between physicians and patients. Something has gone terribly wrong.

We often hear it said that America has the best health care system in the world. I believe that is true, not just because of the money we put into our system or the high-tech machines that help us perform everyday miracles, but because of something even more important—the doctor-patient relationship, which depends on two related freedoms.

In that relationship, as we have long recognized it, the patient is free to choose his or her doctor and facility. This freedom to choose forms the foundation of our market economy and our very nation. True freedom to choose breeds self-correction in the health care marketplace just as in other marketplaces.

Second, the doctor, by virtue of what he has learned both academically and in the trenches (and, I hope, by virtue of his resulting wisdom), earns the freedom to make medical decisions—not just the intellectual authority but the *moral authority* to care for patients. Where a patient's well being is concerned, the combination of the patient's input and the doctor's expertise should make his decision inviolate.

So-called managed care, as it is already evolving even without government intervention, is severely altering the doctor-patient relationship, transforming what can be a very special personal interaction into a business transaction. It is usurping the doctor's decision-making power, forcing diagnostic and treatment decisions to be made by a third party whose central concern is cost.

How could we as a country have come to this point? Is it the medical profession's fault? Perhaps in our occasional haste, our frequent arrogance, our all-too-visible wealth, we doctors have alienated our patients to the point where they will sacrifice the physician-patient relationship.

# Disrobe Completely

Perhaps we drifted apart because the doctor-patient relationship is necessarily one-sided. We physicians are privy to all manner of intimacies gleaned from a patient's health history, but the patient rarely hears anything about the physician's private trials and tribulations. We learn something about the person you are and what has brought you to this moment, but you learn little about who we are and what shaped us.

Some aspects of the health care system are in dire need of reform—but some of the proposed "cures" would destroy the greatest health care system the world has ever seen. As we seek to alter the health care system in America, we should heed the Hippocratic aphorism, *Primum non nocere*, meaning, "First, do no harm."

I want to talk about how to change the system later, but that is just one of my reasons for writing this book. I also want to talk about something that entirely escaped the seminar speaker, Mr. Goatee, and seems to be missing from the debate over reform.

I want to communicate something of the essence of what it is to be a physician. More than any direct argument I can make against managed care, which will *show* you, not just tell you, why it is a grave error to allow the usurpation of the physician's moral and clinical authority by any outside agency.

Now, it would be impractical for a doctor to take up a patient's valuable time during an office-visit to tell his own life story or complain about the new hurdles that complicate a doctor's work today. But estrangement is usually born of misinformation, as are prejudice and envy and violence. If the public is misinformed about the physician in general and about the ways in which managed care is already affecting the quality of their care, then we as doctors should strive to make them better informed.

In this book, you will gain a better understanding of what is involved in becoming a doctor. I also want to share with you the paradox of the doctor-patient relationship. While the patient comes to the doctor in need of his scientific expertise and guidance, it is you, the *patient,* who teaches the vital courses in humanity that supplement the doctor's science. The physician's training coupled with these life lessons puts the physician in the best position to help you make decisions about your health care.

You will also get a glimpse of the frustrations and ultimately the danger of grossly restricting—and finally removing—the doctor's decision-making authority and limiting the patient's freedom to choose a doctor. If we destroy the physician-patient relationship, the very heart of American medicine, our society will be traveling a perilous road indeed.

Finally, you'll be able to consider some possible solutions to the system's very real problems. Unlike the remedies of managed competition, these proposed solutions neither destroy the physician's effectiveness and desire nor restrict the patient's ability to choose his or her own caregiver.

All of the following narratives are true. Some of the names of people and institutions were changed in the interest of privacy. You will find some of these stories sad, some funny, some poignant, and some gruesome, but all played their parts in my development as a physician.

I hope this book helps you understand physicians better and learn that the best doctors become what they are by listening to patients. I've tried to listen. Here is what I've learned.

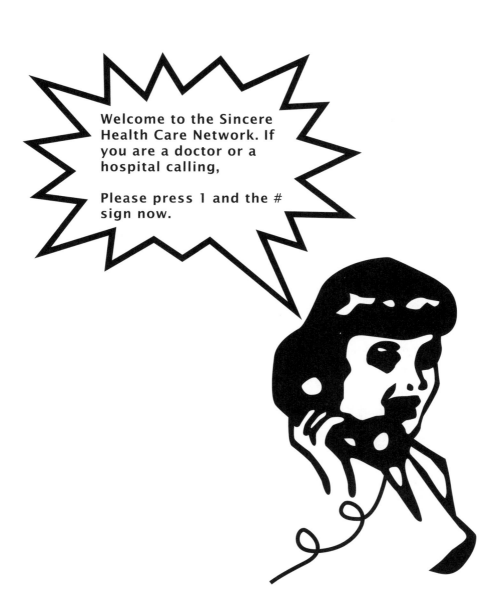

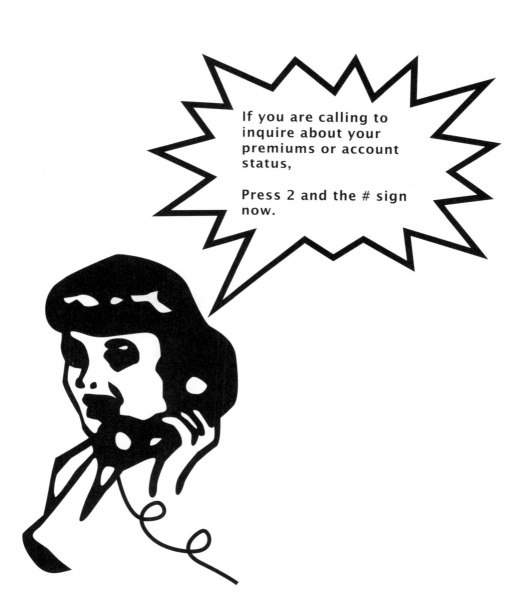

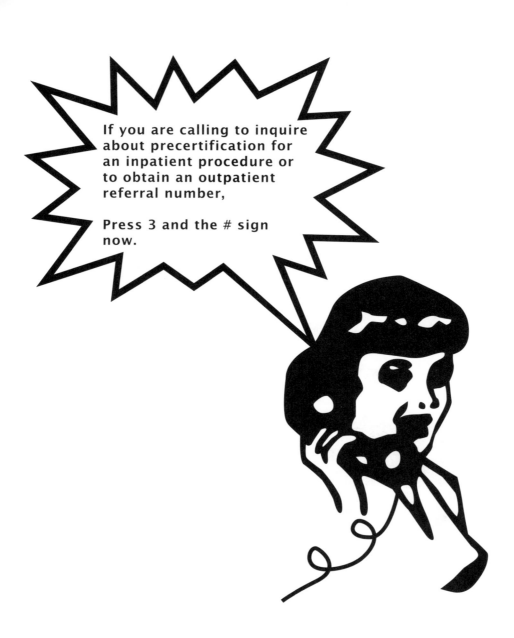

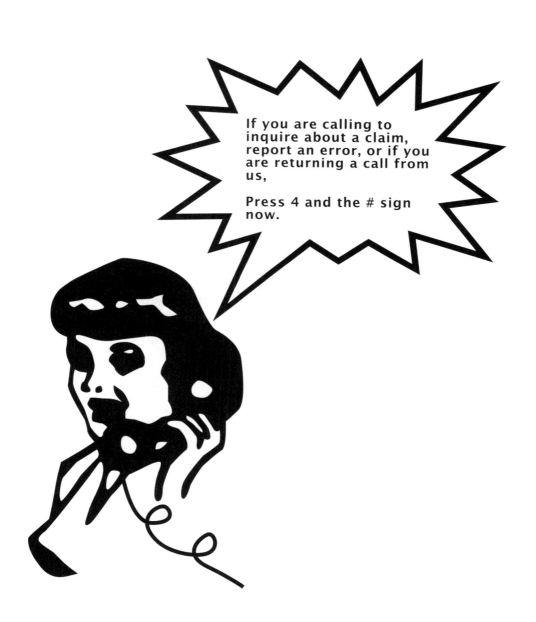

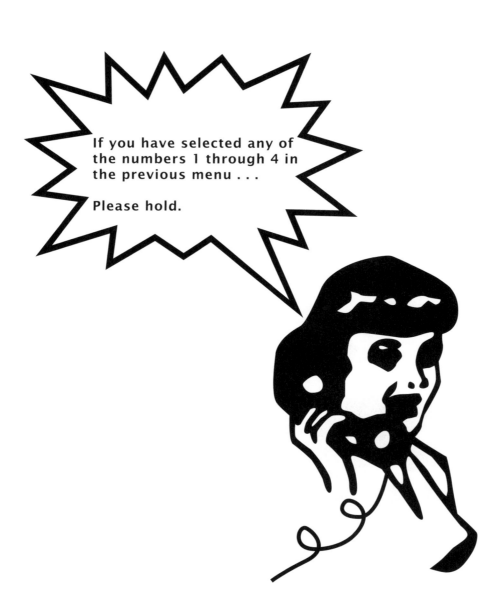

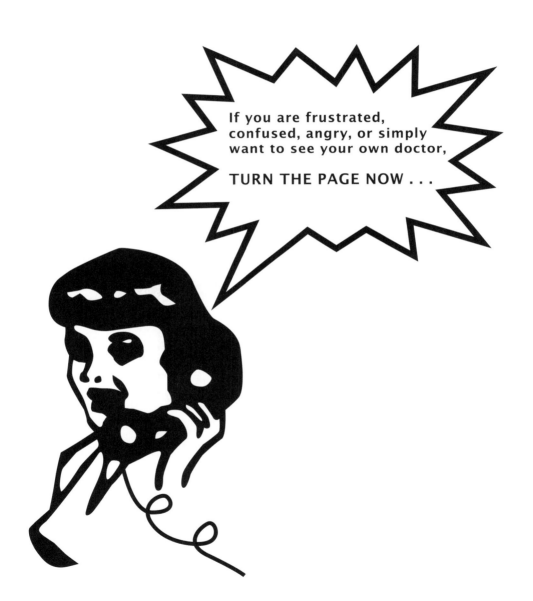

"Seeing much, suffering much, and studying much; these are the three pillars of learning."

—Benjamin Disraeli

# Part I

# Disrobe Completely:
## Naiveté

*While in college, I had almost no concept of what might be involved in medical school above and beyond diligent study. My life from birth to about twenty-one did very little to prepare me for the bizarre experiences I would have while training to be a physician.*

*Looking back on those years, I now realize that some of those experiences shaped the course of future events for me—in fact, they shaped the person that I am. All physicians have similar anecdotes, the war stories one used to hear in physicians' lounges before managed care and medical-legal issues came to dominate the conversation.*

*The lessons begin very early on. They plant the seeds of compassion. They make it possible to suffer together with the patient, in the literal sense of the word* compassionate. *These lessons often contribute more to the future doctor's character than to his fund of knowledge. But it is that character that is the foundation of the physician-patient relationship. In turn, that relationship combined with scientific knowledge puts the physician in the best position to make the decisions that most benefit those patients whose sacred trust he has sworn to uphold.*

# Boldly in Red

---

*Until recently, all medical school candidates had to be in the top 1–5%
of their undergraduate classes. While remaining in this elite group
may seem a substantial challenge in and of itself, most of us left high
school pretty sure of our abilities. All of us were by definition at the top
of our high-school classes and saw no reason why that should change
at the college level.*

*What many of us did not realize is that a lot of those students we left
in the academic dust had never intended to go on to college, so beating them to the finish line was a pretty hollow victory. Furthermore,
many private universities had a way of concentrating the best and the
brightest within their hedges. In short, many of us who would eventually enter medical school were about to have our initial experience
with real competition, and first prize was a lesson in humility.*

---

A perfectly good number really, seventeen—could be good as the chapter number, the number of years since I considered thirty-five to be "old," the age at which the opposite sex was an all-consuming interest, the number of billions that the federal government borrows in a month, the number of games the Dallas Cowboys won in the 92–93 season, the age of my Siamese cat, or any of a myriad of other things.

It is not, however, a particularly good number to have written boldly in red across the top of one's first chemistry test at Rice University.

# Boldly in Red

Now the public perception of physicians may have changed in many ways over the last thirty or forty years, but in some ways, it remains unaltered. In general, most would agree that medical doctors are not dummies. Admittedly, some may have the bedside manner of Bobby Knight, but they're not supposed to be stupid. Even your average high-school student knows that you're not supposed to see a number like seventeen written on anything you ever do, if, in fact, you wish to one day have the initials "MD" after your name.

In short, racking up a seventeen was not a step in the proverbial right direction. But before you conclude that if in fact I was making seventeens on my freshman chemistry tests, perhaps I should not be the one to focus an argon laser in your pelvic cavity, a little background information is warranted.

Rice University's incoming freshman class of 1974 was over 70% National Merit Scholars and over 60% valedictorians. Although only salutatorian in my highly regarded private high school, I could at least lay claim to a National Merit Scholarship. I had placed out of biology, calculus, and English, and was taking chemistry only because I knew that inorganic, then organic, then biochemistry would be required by most medical schools. (I wasn't convinced at this point that I wanted to be a physician, but I wanted to leave all the doors open.) In short, I thought, as did most of the other Rice students, that I was pretty hot stuff academically.

It took exactly nine class days for Rice to make clear that "hot stuff" was a relative term. (*Top Gun* fans—you will recall that Commander Metcalf unceremoniously cleaned Maverick's plow on their first hop over the desert.) Lo and behold, there were people from all over this country with considerably more cerebral firepower than *moi*.

Seventeen. *Seventeen*? Of course, at first I assumed this was the percentage of questions that I had gotten incorrect. Well, that's not so bad . . . Wrong, *mon ami*! Next I assumed that the test would be graded on a curve. Wrong yet again, *mon cher*! In the vernacular, I had flunked it—"screwed the pooch," I believe is the immortal term used by astronaut Gus Grissom after he allegedly let his Mercury space capsule sink to the bottom of the Pacific.

There was some consolation in my discovery that 17% was the third-highest grade in the class. It remained, however, my first academic failure. Not unlike many premed students, in fact, it was the first time in my life that I had received a grade other than an A. (Uh, except for the C I received in—and this is the God's honest truth—handwriting in the third grade.)

This may seem silly to you non-anal-retentive, noncompulsive types, but we premeds saw it as a big deal at the time. You just don't get seventeens. It just flat out does not happen. Denial, remorse, fear, anger, etc., all apply here. Elisabeth Kubler-Ross, author of *On Death and Dying*, would have put this somewhere between losing your spouse and children beneath an overturned cement truck and possibly the annihilation of life as we know it in a nuclear holocaust. Your whole life flashes before your eyes. Forget being a doctor. Forget being an engineer. Forget the possibility of a lucrative life as a small animal vet. Hell, with a seventeen on your record, would a law school even take you?

Well, time heals all wounds, and as I flunked tests in multiple other disciplines, I began to feel much better. This was clearly part of the plan. If it was intended to catch students' attention and get their noses to the grindstone, then we were all down to the cartilage in a matter of weeks.

But like so many other experiences that seem like disasters at the time, this event also shaped the future physician. A little humility goes a long way with colleagues and patients alike. Rice University and that chemistry professor had made a contribution to the humility fund right from the git-go.

Humility, of course, has long been viewed as an essential virtue of the well-rounded character. Ben Franklin added it to his list of virtues to be actively attained in his autobiography. In fact, he did so well with it personally that he reports being "quite proud of my humility."

# Hither and Yonder

---

*Other than television and their own limited encounters with emergency rooms for broken arms and the like, most college students have no exposure to medicine at all. Often, their introduction to the real world of medicine involves a job that offers limited contact with doctors, nurses, technicians, and patients.*

*Some students work as orderlies or clerks. I got an unusual job with an extraordinary mentor, and I learned that a slipshod approach to my job might have put the technician and physician out of work and killed the patient. That in turn taught me the meaning of the word* responsibility.

---

Yonnie. In a roundabout way, Yonnie was responsible for the tremendous blow to my forehead that I received at about 4:30 a.m. on that particular Monday morning.

The more direct cause lay in my position at the time. I was lying beneath the steel desk with my head no more than six feet from the cow theoretically under surveillance. Sleep had been my companion for only about an hour since my last readings. Suddenly something struck the sole of my left foot, jarring me awake and instantaneously propelling me into a sitting position.

Unfortunately, the desk did not quite allow adequate clearance for the sitting position, and thus, the fierce blow to my head occured only microseconds after my foot had been similarly insulted. Needless to say, I uttered several expletives, college students being particularly adept at this form of expression. I slid myself out from under the desk and looked straight up at my assailant. Even more unfortunately, the guilty party was my employer, an extremely well-known six-foot-six-inch cardiothoracic surgeon.

"Who the heck's watching my cows?" he snapped. I didn't think this was the proper time to remind Dr. Cooley that they weren't technically *his* cows. After all, it was 4:30 a.m. But if he wanted to make rounds on the cows before the people, that was certainly his prerogative.

If you're at all confused, add to the scenario that this is taking place on the third floor of the Texas Heart Institute in Houston, Texas, in November 1977. I was a premed student at the prestigious Rice University across the street, trying to earn a few extra bucks in the total artificial heart (TAH) program. This TAH program, among others like it, was continuing the work of many investigators, which would eventually lead to the placement of a permanent artificial heart in Dr. Barney Clark at the University of Utah in 1982. That procedure, and in fact all open-heart procedures, evolved from the pioneering work of Dr. Michael DeBakey. Dr. DeBakey had, in 1932, invented the central component to the heart-lung bypass machine. His later work at Baylor College of Medicine in conjunction with the Rice Biomedical Engineering Department led to a temporary mechanical-assist device, or partially artificial heart, implanted as early as 1963 and subsequently refined in the late 1960s.

My job was to take the Swan Ganz catheter (tube with sensors in the great vessels and chambers of the heart) recordings, administer antibiotics, feed, water, and otherwise nurture two cows whose natural hearts had been replaced with plastic ones that operated pneumatically. (Prior to Barney Clark, there were a large number of less famous cows.)

By day I was a mild-mannered biology major at Rice, but by night I was the phantom technician upon whose shoulders the success or failure of the TAH program firmly rested. Several centers around the world were involved in such research, but the one with which we competed most directly was a very successful group out in Utah.

The Utah folks had calves (little cows, for non-Texans) living for hundreds of days and actually outgrowing their hearts! Our moos had a nasty tendency to die of sepsis or to be sacrificed, as I understood it at the time, in the interest of drug studies for companies who in large part funded the research. We all kinda thought the guys in Utah had an unfair advantage. They were going strictly for longevity records, while our cows had many more holes in their chests for hoses and IVs and therefore many more opportunities for infection while we studied all kinds of drug effects. Nonetheless, longevity counted, and college students who slept on the job did little to advance the cause.

As it happened, when Denton Cooley caught me snoozing, he was most forgiving and allowed me to rise to my feet and fill him in on the night's events. During my stint that night I learned not only cardiopulmonary physiology, as usual, but also one of my first little lessons about self-discipline. Errors in drug administration or readings could lead to faulty data or worse, the premature loss of a cow. That could translate into millions of dollars of lost grant money, which could in turn mean that people lost their jobs, which down the road could mean that sick people lost their lives. All of a sudden I was thankful the good doctor hadn't taken my sleepy head off.

Oh yes, Yonnie. Yonnie is short for "Yonder" as in "Hither and Yonder." These were the Harlequin Great Danes belonging to Dr. Norman, who was actually in direct charge of the TAH program. Yonnie spent her nights in the third floor lab as security and sometimes companion. She liked the couch. So did I, but Yonnie weighed 180 pounds and when she stood on her hind legs, she put her forepaws on my shoulders and looked down at me. Her growl was something like the sound of a Russian T-72 tank maneuvering over a berm just before crushing you into oblivion. She got the couch. I slept on the floor beneath the desk.

# Weight by History

*My first experiences with human patients took place only a few hundred yards from the cows in the Texas Heart Institute. Big county emergency rooms are not only the salvation of many of our nation's trauma victims but also the proving grounds for our physicians-in-training. As such, the medical student comes in contact with family tragedies for the first time with truths that are often stranger than fiction. The following really occurred and taught me that there is often no dignity in death unless we make it so.*

The first two years of medical school are largely didactic and are spent either in a lecture hall or a laboratory of some sort. However, if you wanted an early taste of this doctor stuff, you could work for nothing in the emergency room at night and thus fill the gobs of free time you had available when you eliminated sleep from your agenda. My roommate Ed and I volunteered.

County ERs are the crossroads for every bizarre type of human that you could envisage with a very fertile imagination. Add alcohol, drugs, impatience, sometimes filth, and often animosity, and you have the recipe for some very atypical occurrences. My second night ever in the ER at Ben Taub, a county hospital affiliated with Baylor College of Medicine in Houston, was the setting for this little tragicomedy.

# Weight by History

Medical students at my level were essentially worthless to everyone—doctors, nurses, orderlies, and medical technicians. Why? Because we didn't know our ass from a hole in the ground; that's why. We lacked any and all knowledge that might be considered even remotely useful in a big city ER.

So we were asked to talk to patients who had been waiting for at least ten hours. These patients could be easily identified by looking for those who had not suffered a gunshot wound to the head or chest or for those without protruding knife handles. Some of these moderately sick people were mildly perturbed by the number of shift changes they had witnessed while waiting to be seen.

That particular night I was instructed by one of the residents to take the history of the man in room 4 with chest pain. I quickly ran by this small room on my way to X-ray to complete a previously assigned task, intending to peek around the curtain across the doorway and inform the hapless gentleman that someone would be with him in a moment. At a glance, I saw no one in the room, just a pair of shoes on the bed.

I delivered the films to X-ray and returned in three to four minutes. To my astonishment, the shoes on the bed turned out, on closer inspection, still to contain their owner. The patient had fallen over backwards, off the gurney, and was now in an inverted jackknife position (for you divers) or just flat crumpled upside down on the floor between the gurney and the wall.

I called down the hall for help and then tried to reach the stricken man. The gurney had been forced away from the wall by the patient's backflip and was now firmly wedged between an inset column and the door frame. Undaunted, I climbed onto the gurney to peer down at the victim. That's when I clearly understood we had a very serious problem on our hands. This man must have weighed 400 pounds. (In point of fact, 468 pounds, according to the triage nurse's record of his "weight by history.") While he was poorly illuminated in his present locale, he nevertheless looked too damned blue in my uneducated opinion.

# Disrobe Completely

Because I was the first to discover this unfortunate situation, others were willing to designate me some proprietary interest in the case and thus elected me to crawl under the gurney and hold an oxygen mask to the man's face. I could find no pulse, but then again, I knew very little about where to look. Two residents tried to force the gurney to an angle where it could be extricated, but they failed. They then tried to lift it straight up so that the man might flop, as it were, into a lying position and then be dragged out from under the gurney. This likewise failed and, in fact, worsened the situation in that the man's legs became entangled in the far side's lowered arm rail.

Needless to say, this massively obese gentleman was not doing well. CPR was not physically possible due to his entrapment and would in all likelihood have been ineffectual even if he had been lying on the trauma table. About this time, the room was blossoming with an unbearable odor. Apparently everyone but me knew that this came from the patient and did not suggest a favorable short-term prognosis. In fact, the man was quite dead, but I just couldn't believe it. True, at this point, he looked dead enough. But in death there is usually some sense of dignity, is there not?

Perhaps you think me callous to include this anecdote. But all physicians have found themselves in similar black-humor situations during their training, and such situations do play a role in shaping their demeanor.

The incident had another meaning for me. This was the first person I had ever witnessed dying. I didn't sit at my great-grandmother's bedside as her life ebbed away, never saw an automobile accident, never found myself at the scene of a drowning or any of a thousand more common scenarios in which people pass away. No, I had to see my first death as an acute myocardial infarction in an inverted 468-pound man wedged in a position where we couldn't help him. He wasn't trapped in the cab of his overturned pickup waiting on the Jaws of Life to cut him free; he was stuffed between a gurney and a wall in the emergency room, positioned such that absolutely nobody could help him.

# Weight by History

They had to cut away the door frame with a fire ax to get him out.

I remember clearly going with the resident to see this man's family in the waiting room. Thank God he had no children, but his parents, brother, and wife were all there anxiously awaiting any news. They were huge. They looked just like him. He was here, they told us, for an ingrown toenail. No, he'd never had chest pain to their knowledge. The resident informed them of the forty-six-year-old man's death. Compassion in this case and attention to the importance of some dignity in passing included not elaborating on the exact circumstances of his demise.

# Toe Tag

*The dissection of a cadaver is a strange and unique experience that leaves a medical student with indelible images and a perspective denied the rest of humanity. It is perhaps only in retrospect that we recognize what we have really learned. True, we learn the details of what a marvelous machine the human body is. But we also learn—through its stark absence—that the soul is who we are. When we treat our living patients, it is perhaps their difference from the cadaver, not their similarity, that guides our decision making.*

As I have suggested already, most of the first two years of medical school involves taking notes and asking questions in a lecture hall. There is, however, some laboratory work. Laboratory work, huh? You visualize glass beakers, Bunsen burners, etched and stained countertops and sinks, bad odors, and just a hint of the gorgeous day outside peeking in through the filthy windows, right? Well, you get partial credit for the bad odors.

Try thirty naked, dripping, slippery dead people, reeking of formalin, all lying on metal tables. Now imagine hacking away at one of those cadavers for six months.

Mind you, before walking into this lab for the first time, all of us were fairly close to being normal people. By that I mean the only dead people we had seen were impeccably dressed in open caskets, and they were usually someone we had held dear. Of course, some of us, myself included, had never even seen the well-dressed, well-preserved deceased loved one. Now we were about to learn that medical school was more than notetaking in an auditorium.

None of us had a clue as to what to expect. I clearly remember walking in and seeing the gleaming metal tables and wondering when and where the actual cadavers came into play. There was the expected skeleton hanging in the corner by the blackboard. There was Carl Harvey, PhD, whom we had already come to love as perhaps the most outstanding teacher of the basic science curriculum, standing by the blackboard and waving our four-person groups into position at the assigned, numbered stations. The combination of the odor in its eye-watering intensity with the overhead fluorescents (the sole source of illumination) gave the fourth-floor lab the appearance of a large basement somewhere in Transylvania.

Logic, of course, would dictate that the sun be allowed in such a grim place and maybe even a modicum of fresh air from time to time. Instead, the windows were blacked out with tar paper. No one ever really explained why. Presumably this was done for privacy. Perhaps it was so that any forty-foot-tall relatives of the deceased wouldn't stand a chance of being inadvertently offended? We were to learn, of course, that since morgues are invariably located in the cellar, the interior decorating of this fourth-floor lab would make us feel right at home later in our careers.

My lab partners were Ed, my roommate; Jane, a remarkably attractive blonde (remarkable particularly since she was a fellow Rice alum, and at Rice the admissions process apparently was stacked against pretty girls); and Mark, a handsome Italian-type whose last name just happened to match that of a nationally known mafia figure recently boarded at the government's expense. On that first day, we donned our black aprons and awaited further instructions.

Dr. Harvey informed us that we would be dissecting our cadaver in the order in which neophytes like us could best assimilate information, i.e., easy stuff first. Well, "easy" on a very fat, old, dead lady like ours was definitely extremities first and upper prior to lower. He also informed us that these bodies were donated to the medical school either by their owners or their families. It was only common decency that their names not be revealed, but their causes of death could be ascertained by perusing the computer printout by the lab door.

Then it was time to raise our cadavers from the depths. The tabletops slid open, and several turns of the crank brought our specimens slowly to the surface. (I knew I'd seen this movie before.) The excess formaldehyde sloshed loudly back to the bottom of the metallic table. Some of the less hardy had their eyes closed at this point, anticipating that their donated cadaver would probably have a less pleasing appearance than Aunt Sarah had at the Eternal Rest Funeral Parlor. They needn't have worried because the donors rose to the surface zipped into thirty identical black body bags. (*Why?* you might ask. Well, obviously to keep the smaller parts that were later to be dissected from floating aimlessly and inaccessibly beneath the largely perforated metal sheet that actually rose to support the bodies. Why black? Well, it matched the windows, the aprons, and, initially, the mood.)

I don't recall which of us had the honor of making the first incisions, but I do recall thinking during the process that perhaps I had made a very serious error in career choice. Somehow I knew that at 10:00 a.m. on a Monday there were very few TI engineers or General Electric marketing people immersed in similar tasks.

Despite the ghastly appearance of our specimen, with her yellowish-grey, slippery skin the texture of shoe leather, her few wisps of grey hair, the incredible weight of her obese, rigid extremities, and that overpowering odor, we decided she would have to have a name. "Our cadaver" was not descriptive enough and in fact not worthy of this specimen which was not so long ago the repository of a soul. While others named their cadavers in ways that might easily distinguish them from their twenty-nine colleagues (I will not here enumerate the anatomically related designations at which this group of fertile young minds was able to arrive), we had the misfortune to discover our cadaver's overlooked toe tag. The computer printout had already enlightened us to the age and cause of death (sixty-seven and myocardial infarction, or heart attack—big surprise, I might add) but the tag also revealed her name: Janice Cheops.

Now it was extremely difficult, while looking at her in this condition, to believe that even distant relatives of hers could have descended from the ancient Egyptian emperors suggested by her surname. Accordingly, the four of us simply adopted the name Janice for our cadaver.

Over the course of the next six months, Janice taught us much about the human condition as well as the human body. Obesity became much more of a negative reinforcment for our own health habits, as her liquefying fat made dissection of her corpse infinitely more difficult and disgusting than that of the emaciated old cadaver at the next table over, for example. The carbonization of her lungs by cigarette tar, the cholesterol plaque in her major arteries, the cirrhotic changes of her liver all served as potent memorials to the dangers of smoking, overeating, overdrinking, and underexercising.

After half a year, Janice had become as integral a part of our daily lives as running before work or the minimum three daily showers required to survive the summers in Houston. She was even losing weight gradually, although not via the usual route employed by the living. After removal of the skin came the fat, vessels, muscles and tendons, and finally the bones themselves.

The crowning achievement, if you'll excuse the expression, was the opening of the skull, removal of the brain, and study of the attachments of the cranial nerves and associated vasculature—a process difficult enough to make one wonder exactly how someone could have just misplaced President Kennedy's brain. We opened the cranium with a bone saw and lifted off the top of the skull, which then looked just like a Jewish yarmulke.

It was at this juncture that many of us sneaked into the lab on the last Saturday before the final exams and obtained a memento of the good times we'd all had together. We used a 35 mm Minolta set on timer to create a portrait of Janice in the sitting position surrounded by her weight-loss management team. Mark, Ed, Jane, and I put on our best smiles while being literally supportive of our teacher.

Now, doing this was strictly against medical-school policy. It would be nothing short of disastrous should such a photo ever be seen by the cadaver's loved ones. It would be not only embarrassing and even cruel, but—who knows—the family may have donated their relative's money in addition to their relative! We felt sufficiently secure, however, in the knowledge that Janice was, well, quite frankly, unrecognizable, despite our best efforts to patch her up for the shot. (The editor has recommended that I not include the photograph here, and I have deferred to her judgment.)

The reader may think this callous, even bizarre. I think of it now as a way of coping with an experience that I daresay is shared by less than 0.01% of the population. Each day, we had to slice into what, for all intents and purposes, was another human being, a creature who had known reason and laughter and tears, and yet our training required that we treat her as no more than a bag of veins, tendons, and muscles—inert meat. We needed humor to lighten the burden. The humor was a shield against the strangeness of it all.

The true desecration was not our humor, but the repeated damage that these corpses' former owners had inflicted on themselves. Our Janice was in all senses an empty shell. Her body may once have been a temple, but when the soul departed, it became only a testimony to its defilement, however unintentional, in life.

The images which we physicians take away with us from those anatomy laboratories remain vivid for the rest of our lives. If we fail to see the damage we inflict on our own bodies through lack of sleep, lousy diets, inordinate stress, alcohol, drugs, and cigarettes, perhaps some of us will at least be able to see what those choices are doing to you by remembering our "Janices."

# Aequanimitas

---

*All professions have their own unique pressures. With few exceptions, however, allowing that pressure to affect your performance adversely leads to consequences only for the individual. Physicians, not unlike airline pilots, can kill people when the pressure gets to them.*

*Some have criticized formal medical-education programs in which medical students and residents work as many as 120 hours per week. They may criticize the public humiliation many students and residents are exposed to in the course of case presentations to more senior physicians. But these are the things that teach the value of evenness under pressure. When you're under the knife, wouldn't you rather know that your physician has been tested by the most adverse physical and emotional circumstances and survived intact?*

---

A *equanimitas* is both an ancient Latin word and the title of a collection of addresses presented at various places and in various times by the great William Osler, BT, MD, FRS, professor of medicine at Oxford and honorary professor of medicine at Johns Hopkins University. Specifically, Osler delivered the eponymous address of the collection as a valedictory to the University of Pennsylvania Medical School on May 1, 1889.

*Aequanimitas* and its English cognate, *equanimity*, denote evenness of mind, especially under stress. It is, as Osler points out, regrettable but necessary that a physician, in order to be possessed of equanimity, must distance himself from the emotions that surround the horrors with which he has chosen to deal for the rest of his life, or go mad.

> In the first place, in the physician or surgeon, no quality takes rank with imperturbability . . . Imperturbability means coolness and presence of mind under all circumstances, calmness amid storm, clearness of judgment in moments of grave peril. It is the quality which is most appreciated by the laity though often misunderstood by them . . . and the physician who has the misfortune to be without it, who betrays indecision and worry, and who shows that he is flustered and flurried in ordinary emergencies, loses rapidly the confidence of his patients.

Professor Osler goes on to say the following:

> . . . From its very nature this precious quality is liable to be misinterpreted, and the general accusation of hardness, so often brought against the profession, has here its foundation. Now a certain measure of insensitivity is not only an advantage, but a positive necessity in the exercise of a calm judgment, and in carrying out delicate operations. . . . Cultivate then gentlemen, such a judicious measure of obtuseness as will enable you to meet the exigencies of practice with firmness and courage, without, at the same time, hardening "the human heart by which we live.". . . The mental equivalent to this bodily endowment (imperturbability), is the watchword, *Aequanimitas*.

# Disrobe Completely

If a physician in fact achieves this evenness under pressure, this imperturbability, he may then have some hope of succeeding in his field. Without it, first his patients' confidence fails, and next, of course, his confidence in his own capabilities crumbles as well. All of this probably seems self-evident. But what you might not appreciate is the extreme situations in which this quality of *aequanimitas* becomes absolutely essential.

I use as an illustration something that happened to a surgical resident and friend of my brother while I was in my second year of basic science. While not, thank God, a firsthand participant, I include this as one of the experiences that colored my medical education.

The resident was working in the county emergency room in the X-ray annex to one of the trauma rooms. The patient lying on the X-ray table was bleeding profusely from an obvious gunshot wound to the upper left thigh. The thigh itself was swollen and discolored. The resident was in the midst of passing a large bore catheter into the groin to be used for injecting radio-opaque dye, a so-called angiogram. The purpose of this test was to ascertain if in fact the femoral artery had been severed by the bullet, which had passed completely through the leg.

The patient was a big man dressed in black sweatpants (now opened up the leg with scissors), and a bloody, filthy, formerly white T-shirt. He was semiconscious, rolling his head back and forth, and moaning. Other than the female technician across the table from the resident, the only people in the room were two plainclothes police officers positioned near the top of the bed. While the resident was aware that the man was in custody, he was not aware of the crime he had allegedly committed.

Just after the catheter was successfully threaded, while the resident and the technician were watching the fluoroscope monitor at the foot of the bed, one of the police officers inquired as to whether his prisoner "would make it." Before the surgeon could respond, the small tiled room reverberated with a tremendous explosion. The technician and the surgical resident jumped up, covered their ears, and turned to see the two men in suits wrestling a uniformed officer to the floor. The patient was no longer moaning. In fact the better portion of his skull and contents were splattered across the leaden glass wall separating X-ray from trauma. According to my brother, the resident kept his cool, never missing a beat, and answered the officer's question: "Evidently not."

It turned out that the patient had murdered the uniformed officer's partner of eight years. While the resident was obviously shaken by the incident, he did not collapse to the floor in a whimpering heap or run from the room screaming. This truly is imperturbability on a herculean scale! Not surprisingly, the resident later became a trauma surgeon.

You may ask how anyone could be so unfeeling as to respond to this situation in this way. I ask you: how could an effective physician respond in any other way?

There will be many other incidents detailed in the following pages which illustrate this elusive *Aequanimitas*. Many are less gruesome and more poignant, but all involve a doctor's developed ability to separate his natural human responses from the situation and control his temperament and actions.

# The Strong Survive

*Mental and emotional stress are facts of life in the training of the phy-sician from medical school on—and some of that stress is deliberately inflicted in a ritual some may see as cruel. But the doctor-in-training must learn to function on the spot, right that second, sometimes with a life hanging in the balance. Though this trial-by-fire can be painful and humiliating, the ritual teaches the future doctor to think and act swiftly and precisely.*

Samuel Johnson once observed that "when a man knows he is to be hanged in a fortnight, it concentrates his mind wonderfully." So does pimping.

Now don't get the wrong idea. Don't picture girls in leather minis and heavy mascara walking the streets while a diamond-studded business man-ager lurks in the shadows. As far as any physician I know can remember, the derivation of the term "pimping" is unrelated to the oldest profession.

In the world of medical training, "pimping" refers to the painful ritual wherein one person (usually the ordinate) asks another person (usually the sub-ordinate) a question or series of questions to which there are no specific right answers, thus forcing the subordinate to publicly humiliate himself and either collapse on the floor in a sobbing heap or quietly but noticeably wet his pants.

The medical student is first introduced to pimping during study sessions with a roommate or some other classmate. Those of us who were successful at this game recognized its essential role early on in the entire portal process. At every level of a doctor's education, from basic sciences to clinical rotations to internship and residency, he or she must successfully negotiate these rites of passage, and the guardian of the gate is usually called a "pimper."

The highest ranking students quickly figured out how to survive the ongoing pimping ritual that is medical school: don't think—memorize. If you could memorize the Manhattan phone book over a weekend (and many of us could), you had it made in the shade—thanks in part to cramming sessions propelled by what we called the "V-2 rocket," Vivarin. Why waste time preparing and actually drinking thirty or forty cups of coffee if you can get the equivalent boost more quickly and easily in capsule form? No illegal amphetamines for us, no sir. We just totally wired ourselves on the V-2 rocket, and we were off, stretching our synapses to the breaking point with vast loads of factoids.

What? Trouble remembering that histamine breaks down into methyl histamine, methylimidazole acetic acid, imidazole acetic acid riboside, imidazole acetic acid and acetylhistamine? Pop another V-2, and read it again while you use your yellow highlighter. (Eventually, every line of every medical textbook is highlighted.) Once the task of reading, rereading, and highlighting was completed, the study mates would combine forces and come up with mnemonics that would help them visualize this mass of detail, for example, this little number for the muscles of the medial thigh:

Say . . . . . . . . . . . . . . . . . . Sartorious
Grace . . . . . . . . . . . . . . . . . Gracilis
Before . . . . . . . . . . . . . . . . Semi-membranosus
Tea . . . . . . . . . . . . . . . . . . Semi-tendinosus

Of course, Vivarin-driven minds sometimes combined the salacious with the utilitarian, producing helpful devices like this one for the bones of the hand:

# Disrobe Completely

She . . . . . . . . . . . . . . . . . Scaphoid

Loved. . . . . . . . . . . . . . . Lunate

Tom's. . . . . . . . . . . . . . . Triquetrum

Piston. . . . . . . . . . . . . . . Pisiform

Tunneling . . . . . . . . . . . . Trapezium

(her) Groove . . . . . . . . . . . Groove of Trapezium

Tightly . . . . . . . . . . . . . . Trapezoid

Clenching . . . . . . . . . . . . Capitate

His . . . . . . . . . . . . . . . . Hamate

Manhood. . . . . . . . . . . . . Metacarpals

Sometimes, however, mnemonics and the V-2 rocket were not enough. Picture yourself in this scenario.

It's 0700 Monday morning. You've been up for the last forty-eight hours on your emergency room rotation as a part of your internship at Anytown's Big County Hospital. Twelve of you, men and women, are packed into a tiny conference room without enough chairs. Some of your compadres are leaning against the walls; some are hiked up onto windowsills. Each of you, in filthy, sweaty scrubs, smells like the Newark city dump—no time for showers in the recent past.

After meager rations of very strong coffee in plastic cups and very stale donuts in paper towels, an impeccably dressed attending surgeon—slightly graying, mustachioed, and much feared—enters the room. In his horn-rim glasses and long white coat, he takes a seat reserved especially for him. Without a preliminary word he says: "Dr. Sawyer?" The room falls deathly quiet. The lion roaming the Serengeti has picked his lame gazelle.

"Yes, sir?" answers an exhausted intern.

"He's lying on the trauma table in the ER. The ambulance crew has just stepped aside. He has one eighteen-gauge antecubital IV in his left arm wide open with lactated Ringer's solution. He is blue. What do you do?"

"I'd begin CPR," says Sawyer confidently.

"Excuse me. You'd do what?"

Again, with slightly less *savoir faire*, "Ah, I'd begin CPR."

"Don't you think you ought to check and see if he's breathing on his own before you decide to do it for him?"

"Well, yeah, I mean, sure. Check for respiration and if there is none, begin CPR."

"Hold it," the professor again. "Aren't we forgetting another tiny little detail, doctor? Perhaps you're interested in his pulse. You remember, cardiac function? The 'c' part in 'CPR'?"

Now every intern knows the basics of CPR. The unsuspecting gazelle expected questions along the line of, "How many milligrams of bretylium per kilo do you give in ventricular fibrillation after lidocaine, epinephrine, and isuprel have failed?"

By now everyone in the room knows what kind of morning it's going to be. This will not be fair pimping. This will be a bloody, ugly affair. "OK! After I check for the absence of pulse, I begin CPR." Dr. Sawyer is somewhat exasperated.

"Oh, so tell me, doctor, you don't think the pulse is all that critical to ascertain?" The sarcasm drips from the surgeon like mucous from the nose of a two-year-old.

"Yes, sir, I think it's important." Sawyer's voice is losing its snap. The gazelle is tiring.

"Well, let's assume you're awake enough, Dr. Sawyer, to initiate CPR, start a central line, get the patient intubated, send off some blood gases, put some EKG leads on, and get a pattern. What you see is the old qrST [normal heart wave patterns] lookin' just fine, but your patient has no pressure and isn't breathing. What are we dealing with? Anyone else?"

Well, every intern there knows the answer. EMD, electromechanical dissociation. But the gazelle on the fringe of the herd is beginning to panic now. He can feel the lion's hot breath on his hindquarters, and he knows it's hopeless. His only hope lies in the rest of the herd drawing the lion's attention.

Not very damn likely. We've seen what kind of a morning this is. This is not a learning morning in the conventional sense. This is a learn-just-exactly-how-low-a-form-of-life-the-intern-is morning. Which means that jumping in with the answer will indeed turn the big cat's attention momentarily, just long enough for him to rip out your throat before returning to finish off the original quarry. "I think that's that disassociated thing . . . sir." Dr. Sawyer's breathing is becoming labored.

The surgeon looks around the room. Suddenly, those plastic cups of cooling coffee seem worthy of intense study. Everyone manages to be looking elsewhere at the critical millisecond of visual intercept. The surgeon is disgusted. "That disassociated thing, doctor? What thing is that exactly?" the surgeon asks with a derogatory smirk.

"I guess it's where the electrical signal is present in the heart, but for whatever reason the pump can't supply a pressure?" Dr. Sawyer looks up fleetingly. Could the big cat's attention be turned elsewhere with a partially correct response? Not a chance.

"How do you help the man, doctor?"

"I'd give him calcium chloride epinephrine and start a dopa drip?" The panicked gazelle turning to make a stand? Does he think that he can dodge the onrushing, tightly wound bundle of pure muscular hellcat?

"Well, Dr. Sawyer, you do that. Nothing happens. Nothing. You're killing him—you know that, don't you? Every second is precious and you're standing around pumping him full of medicines that don't work while he dies. Are you gonna tell his family you were just too sleepy to think of the right approach? Well, are you?"

Only the rattle of the anemic air conditioner can be heard in the room. A few people shuffle to change position. Jesus! How long can this go on?

"No, ah, sir." The big buck is on his side now. Froth bubbles from his mouth. His dusty coat is turned muddy by the sheen of sweat. He furiously throws his head in the air one last time before the crushing jaws close across his neck. "I'd do a paracentesis. Yeah, that's what I'd do. I'd take an eighteen-gauge spinal needle, insert it under the sternum to the left, and aim upwards until I aspirated the pericardial fluid causing his tamponade!"

"And what is tamponade, Dr. Sawyer?"

"Well, the fluid trapped in the sac around the heart. The fluid compresses the heart and makes it an ineffective pump."

"So you'd put a needle in it and drain it?"

"Uh, yes, sir."

"Oh, that would be excellent, Dr. Sawyer. Excellent. Then you wouldn't be guilty of incompetence. I'd say you'd be guilty of murder. Murder by proactive stupidity. Remember when you were supposed to have intubated your patient? You were supposed to listen for breath sounds, remember? You wouldn't have heard them on the right while breathing for him with the ambu bag. Why not?"

"You're down a main stem bronchus?" says a new voice from the back. The lion never shifts his gaze from the original prey.

"You people amaze me. First of all, it's the right main stem bronchus that gets intubated accidentally, so that's obviously not the case here. Why don't we have breath sounds, Dr. Sawyer?"

"I . . . I . . . don't know." The razor sharp teeth sink through the loose hide over the windpipe, then rip a huge hunk out of the carcass.

"Ever heard of a tension pneumothorax, people? All this poor bastard needed was for this summa cum laude desk jockey here to put a sixteen-gauge needle in his right chest, bleed off the air in the pleural cavity, kickstart him with a little epi if needed, and then place the chest tube. Well, Dr. Sawyer, it's only

# Disrobe Completely

0723 on a Monday, and you've already killed somebody. How does it feel?"

Dr. Sawyer looks steadily at the floor. His eyes are glistening, his face frozen with humiliation and fury. He doesn't answer as the herd moves on, the surgeon now launching into a didactic covering acid/base balance and calculation of base deficit.

The prey lay in its own gore, flies gathered as the sun approached its zenith. This herd animal learned the hard way that the only protection from this kind of ferocious assault, the worst kind of pimping, was to be sure you knew all, and I mean *all*, the damn answers.

# My Tool

*Physicians deal with some horrible things, including the damage one angry person can do to another in a society where handguns are rampant. I've often wondered why the movies don't show what it's really like after someone has been shot. I don't mean the gore; there's more than enough of that on film. But they don't often show the agony, the writhing, the continuous screaming, or the abject terror.*

*In becoming a physician, I was exposed for the first time to some of these horrors. Up close, you learn the body is all too easily destroyed. But you also learn that the body and the mind are inextricably entwined. Even in the bloody ruins of a gunshot victim's body, the human feelings that give us our identity live on. And regardless of the circumstances that brought this person to these last moments of pain and terror, he can be helped with a kind word—even if it stretches the truth.*

P art of the physician's task involves recognizing the patient as a human being. This means more than merely remembering that your patients have feelings. It also means seeing all your patients as equally deserving of your best efforts to ease their suffering.

I was working again as a volunteer in the emergency department of the county hospital. It was about 1:00 a.m. on a Sunday morning. This was remarkable only in that basic science final exams were beginning on Monday, and I didn't *have* to be in the ER. But I wanted to be there. After all, the patients were the point, not the textbooks. We wanted to be where the action was. We wanted to do the doctor thing as soon as possible. Saturday night was the usual meeting of the "knife and gun club." The Mexican gangs mostly used knives, probably for both cultural as well as financial reasons. The blacks, on the other hand, used guns exclusively.

Well, if you have ever played "rock, paper, scissors," you know that guns beat knives almost every time.

In any event, I was lying across the chest of a particularly exercised black male about twenty years old. I was one of several people trying to keep him on the trauma table while the nurses cut away his jeans to assess the damage he had suffered while exchanging fire with police. My immediate assumption, being an upper-middle-class white boy, was that he must have screwed up big time. The SOB probably deserved whatever he got.

He was thrashing about, foaming at the mouth, jerking his head back and forth, screaming, "My tool, my tool, I gots to know, is my tool all right?"

It was a wonder he could speak at all. The right side of his face was gone, just flat out gone. I remember as clearly as if it were yesterday that I could see all the way down his throat through a hole the size of a softball where his right cheek and jaw should have been. How could he even swallow his own blood and saliva, much less articulate those words? It took a moment for me to even understand what his "tool" was or why he was so upset about that when half his face was gone.

Then the nurses got his pants off, and in turning my head to keep his spittle from my face, I saw why he was disturbed. Most of his upper left thigh was unrecognizable. But even more horrifying than the bloody wreck of his leg was the fact that only shreds of his scrotum and penis remained. As the blood poured from his groin and face and neck, his struggles became weaker. His shouting turned to moaning.

I knew he had been in a fight with the cops, but as he was dying in front of me, I couldn't help thinking what it must be like for him. I was twenty-two. I knew my "tool" certainly played a big part in my future, even if its current role was somewhat diminished by time constraints. Was it really so absurd that he should be more worried about his manhood than the ragged shreds of a face he had left?

I was still lying across his chest. As he weakened I leaned over and shouted in his ear, "It's all right, man. Your tool is totally cool. Shotgun just caught your upper leg is all. You hear me, man? You're okay!"

He grabbed my shoulder with his right arm. His face, or what remained of it, was about six inches from mine. "Thanks, man, thanks a lot."

Those were his last words. He died right there. I got the hell out of the way, and the people who knew what they were doing coded him for a while, but they gave up after about five minutes.

It turned out he was shot while robbing a liquor store. He'd killed an eighteen-year-old Vietnamese girl shortly after the police arrived on the scene. People around the trauma room got a laugh out of his concern for his genitals. Some made comments about how you'd expect that from one of the brothers.

Then an unexpected thing happened to me. I found myself furious with the people making fun of him. I was too young and naive to recognize their defense mechanisms for dealing with this horror, but I knew one thing: this poor bastard shouldn't have died at twenty, no matter what he'd done.

Many years later my father gave me a piece of paper he'd carried in his wallet for fifty-seven years. It was titled the "Sanibel Success Story."

Success is the word for which there could be a thousand definitions. A great many people equate success with money.

The fact is that there are millions of affluent failures and

an equal number of successes who have nothing in the bank.
One definition of success is to win the respect of
intelligent persons and the affection of children, to
earn the approval of honest critics and endure the
betrayal of false friends.

To appreciate beauty, to find the best in others and
to have accomplished a rescued soul.

To have played and lived with enthusiasm and seen with
exultation, to know that even one life has breathed
easier because you have lived.

This is to have succeeded.

These thoughts that my father valued so highly reminded me of this story. This man had deserved my help, no matter his color, his creed, his station, or his actions. I felt sorry for the girl he had killed, but I had no regrets about what I had said to him or done for him.

If for one brief moment before he died, this man had breathed easier because of me, then that was successful medicine.

# Spanish Inquisition

*Now here is a satanic concept worthy of Machiavelli himself. The Spanish inquisitors were no more adept at torture than modern day academicians selected as oral examiners. This is the ultimate rite of passage, the final portal through which many specialists must pass, and thus its inclusion in this section, despite that fact that orals come two years after residency. Just the word "orals" strikes fear and loathing into the hearts of those who have survived to practice medicine in the real world.*

Orals are roughly comparable to thesis defense for a doctoral degree, but the consequences of failure are not the same. Failure on the oral exams in obstetrics and gynecology not only means humiliation for you and your residency program, but also nowadays may mean loss of the right to apply for hospital privileges, alteration of referral status for managed health care plans, reduced reimbursement from those insurers that will still recognize you as a provider—in short, the end of the dream for which you have worked over the last ten grueling years.

Now remember, we're talking about abject terror here. We are not talking about nervousness. We are not talking about apprehension. We are not talking about a little anxiety. We're talking about finding Edgar Allen Poe's telltale heart on the pillow next to you after you switch on the light at three in the morning to investigate a noise in the house.

# Disrobe Completely

Remember also that we are talking about a very select subset of the world's population—a group of men and women who have already been tested more than the average person would be in ten lifetimes. These people already have their medical degrees. They've already completed at least eight years of pimping and been under fire in the trenches for the last four years. These people are not marshmallows. Most have just completed their first two years in practice and, just before that, their tours as chief residents. They are much more accustomed to being the interrogator than the interrogatee.

The torture really begins long before you arrive in the dungeon. The American Board of Obstetrics, Gynecology, and Infertility requires that the physician keep a detailed case list of every delivery and/or operation for the year immediately prior to sitting for the exam. This list must include evidence of adequate exposure to all types of clinical situations. If either the form or content of the list submitted four months prior to the exam is deemed inadequate by some unseen god, you may be refused permission to sit for the exam until the following year. Once you receive notification of acceptance of your case list, family emergencies, deathly illnesses, floods, earthquakes, and nuclear war are all unacceptable excuses for not appearing in the assigned city at the assigned time.

In my case, the assigned city was Chicago. The assigned time was smack dab in the dead of winter. Cold? A bit. Howling gales. Tribes of Eskimos muklukking from one igloo to the next. You know what it feels like to fall through a sea lion's breathing hole into the Arctic Ocean? What about immersing your genitals in a vat of liquid nitrogen? It will freeze your youknowwhats off! That is Chicago in the winter.

As I entered the lobby of the modern high-rise hotel where the orals were to take place, I ran into only one person I knew from Dallas. She had taken her test the day before and was now preparing to leave for the airport. "Absolute piece of cake," she exclaimed. Examiners were pussycats. Don't worry about it!

# Spanish Inquisition

In my extensive test-taking experience, this was an extremely dismal sign. The implication was clear: the exam was a total bitch. So bad in fact, that this relatively bright chick didn't even realize when she'd been wasted! Oh God! Now I was really worried.

The exam is in three parts. Depending on a draw, you begin and then rotate through a) microscope slides, b) kodachromes, and c) case list review. The examiners can ask any question they deem appropriate related to the slide or kodachrome in front of you or to a case chosen from your list.

Now only a truly demented mind could come up with some of these questions and claim they were related to what we had studied. Imagine that the slide concerns the Titanic. You have memorized dates, the number of decks, people, lifeboats, survivors, the name of the captain of the Carpatheia, etc. And here comes the question: "In the cold waters of the North Atlantic, what type of shark are you most likely to encounter?" Arggh.

My first two examiners were men. They asked relatively direct questions about the microscope slides and the kodachromes. True, there were some photos of young men/ladies with ambiguous sexual characteristics, and no one could talk intelligently about them without a review of the appropriate genetics and biochemical pathways immediately before the exam. But there were only a few like that, and I was beginning to wonder after the first two hours if I might *not* end up pumping gas at a Texaco.

Then it happened. I entered another hotel room for my case list review to find a very severe but attractive woman of about forty from Columbia University seated with a clipboard in her lap. She did not look up when I entered the room. I introduced myself, held out my hand, and asked her where she was from. Still not flattering me with even a glance, the examiner castrated me with this: "Have a seat. I don't really think this is the place for social pleasantries." Well, excuuuuuuuuuuuuse me!

The next forty-five minutes were unforgettable to say the least. This doctor dissected me like a cadaver. How, with a list of hundreds of cases, twenty examinees, and probably no time to read the list, could this hellcat zero in on the very few that I wish weren't on there? The laparoscopic ovarian cystectomy, which predated the procedure's popularity by about five years, was used to rip my lungs out. By the time the *kommandant* was through with me, I was scheming about how I might eventually move from the pump to the cash register, then perhaps someday to assistant manager.

I don't know how I managed to check out, get a cab, and find the obscure terminal concourse used for the puddle jumper to Cedar Rapids, Iowa, where I would visit my old medical school roommate. While I waited for the plane at the gate, I called my wife back in Dallas. She deserved to know now that, in light of the limited opportunities for advancement at the Texaco, she would have to go back to work if the kids were going to private school.

I got her on the line and told her the test was fine right up until I met this incredible (while turning) BITCH (now seeing her waiting for the phone directly behind me) who destroyed any hope of a future for the two of us. Now I ask you: Chicago O'Hare, one of the largest, busiest airports in the world, and who's out at gate ZZ-33 waiting for a puddle jumper to Duluth? The catamount from Columbia. Any doubt about my flunking the orals vanished in her tight-lipped smile as she simultaneously recognized me and acknowledged the reference to her personally.

Did the examiners mail in their evaluations? Was there a vote among the three examiners preceded by discussion? Did the inquisitor meet a fiery end just short of the runway in Duluth? Who knows? But some miracle did happen, because six weeks later I received notification by mail. I would not be applying at any local service stations. I had made it!

Now, the not-so-good news was that the American College of Obstetricians and Gynecology (ACOG) decided subsequently that all physicians must recertify (with orals) every ten years or be removed from the college. Which graduating year did they pick as the first that would fall retroactively under these new rules? Mine. My year. You guessed it. I was supposed to be on the line again in 1998. I had thought maybe that time I'd draw New Orleans, Houston, Bogota, anyplace but Chicago in the winter! As it turned out, the American College of Ob/Gyn actually moved to Dallas in the nineties and created annual board certification where the physician can choose to read sixty or so articles each and every year and then take a test over the material. This avoids the exam every ten years and works well for continuing education. I guess even the powers-that-be recognized that orals really ought to be a once-in-a-lifetime experience, albeit now given under the grueling arctic conditions found in Dallas, Texas, each December!

All of us have portals through which we must pass in our lifetime. Some are unavoidable: the death of parents, the ravages of age on our bodies, our children becoming independent and moving away. Some of them are by choice: college entrance exams, graduate-school work, marriage, (and for some, divorce), having children, etc. Oral exams for the physician are technically something he chooses to do but definitely not something he would ever choose to do again. Living through them, however, teaches you priorities. After it's over, you realize that death was not actually as imminent as it had seemed at the time.

A wise person once said, "Don't ever confuse inconvenience with real problems." Isn't that the truth? Next time you think the world's crashing in around you, remember—you could be Afghani, or Kurdish, or a U.S. marine in Iraq, or the relative of one lost there, or you could live in Darfur, or just live in Biloxi, or in short, actually have some real problems.

As the neophyte physician achieves the self-awareness to recognize the portal process for what it is—i.e., a sequence of steps which must be taken but which, if missed, do not represent the end of the world—he moves from *becoming* a doctor to actually *being* a doctor. While he may have a better perspective on his own career path, he is just beginning to understand that now, missed steps can mean the end of the world—for his patient. Part 2 of this book explores the grave responsibilities (pun intended) that go hand in hand with signing the initials "MD" after your name.

"Words of compassion, skillfully administered, are the oldest therapy known to man."

—Louis Nizer

# Part 2

# Put the Gown on So It Opens in Front:

## Experience

*The exhausting, mesmerizing thrill of medical school gives way rapidly—overnight really—to the exhausting new responsibility of internship and residency—four to six years during which the successful physician will earn the moral and clinical authority for medical decision making. Then he or she leaves residency and enters practice or academics as a "real" doctor, someone whose decisions are final and who holds the ultimate responsibility for the patient's care.*

*Well, that's how it was until fairly recently. For the first half of my twenty-five years in medicine, I made diagnostic and therapeutic choices with only these criteria in mind: what would best serve the interests of my patient? What would I do if this were my wife? As a compassionate physician, I suffer with my patients, and I strive to alleviate their suffering as if it were my own.*

*These vignettes are drawn from a time before health care providers existed, a time when doctors delivered care to their patients 24/7, and I was one of them.*

# Not in Kansas Anymore

*Many people suffer from the illusion that American medicine is a clearly definable entity that is essentially uniform from sea to shining sea. Having gone to medical school in one city, done my internship and residency in a second city, and settled in yet another for practice, I know that nothing could be further from the truth. Because medicine is an art and not a science, its practitioners vary widely from one part of the country to the next.*

*Having seen medicine practiced in different ways and in different places, the polished physician has the luxury of choosing from the best of techniques learned—but there's often some culture shock along the way. For instance, if you ask a San Francisco scrub nurse for a peon, she 1) looks as though she hasn't heard you, 2) says, "Say what?" or 3) in a moment of compassion, hands you the* Kelly *and educates you to the instrument's proper name. You could say the same for a* mosquito *in the city by the bay and a* hemostat *in Houston; a* schnit *in San Francisco and a* right angle *in Dallas; a* DeBakey *and a* fine atraumatic, *an* Army-Navy *and an* s-retractor, *a* malleable *and a* ribbon *or* fish, *and on and on, and you get the idea.*

*But the differences run much deeper than medical terminology, extending to the people themselves. From one metropolitan area to another, the patients vary dramatically in their cultural makeup, as I learned in the early eighties when I served an internship in San Francisco, the city that put the multi in multicultural.*

# Not in Kansas Anymore

I t was my first day at San Francisco General Hospital. I didn't even know where the bathrooms were yet. After an all-too-brief orientation, we interns were thrown to the wolves. About 6:00 p.m. I was doing my first delivery as a real live MD. I had delivered several hundred babies as a medical student at Jeff Davis Hospital in Houston (or at least kept them from hitting the floor), but this was my first as an actual doctor.

Cultural variation number one: in 1980 in Houston, patients usually delivered in a very sterile, brightly lit room reminiscent of the standard operating room. In San Francisco, most patients delivered in a Marriott Residence Inn–style room built into the hospital. It had everything but the magic fingers and the coin box. (Okay, I'm *old*! I'm a male gynecologist over fifty—by definition I'm a *gynosaur*.)

OK. I can adapt to this, no problem.

Next difference: in Houston, most women wanted an epidural. Pain was bad. In San Francisco, many women shunned epidurals. Pain was, if not good, at least natural, and drugs (at least these drugs) were bad. Therefore, the typical patient in San Francisco could get very vocal as the pain increased. Naturally.

Finally, picture the brand-new doctor kneeling at the end of the Marriott bed, bending over sideways with a wholly inadequate goose-neck lamp, trying desperately to visualize the torn "virginia" into which he was less than deftly placing sutures. The stirrups to which I had been accustomed were not in evidence, and the patient was forced to try and keep her legs bent at the knee and separated—all this while her pain was inadequately controlled with local anesthetic, and the bed was soaked through with blood, amniotic fluid, urine, and fecal matter.

On that first day, I had forgotten that I was in a city where almost everyone wanted to deliver squatting in Golden Gate Park while chewing alfalfa sprouts. While Mom held her new baby, Dad slipped over to the delivery bed behind me. He quietly removed his shirt. The labor nurse in the room took no notice of him whatsoever. Between stitches, I glanced in his direction and witnessed the first of many cultural exchanges and revelations that were to broaden my horizons during the next four years. Dad reached into the plastic basin on the instrument table and removed the placenta. Carefully rearranging the membranes so that the maternal side of the disc would be exposed, he proceeded to wipe the bloody organ all over his chest and face. Luckily, I was speechless.

When I regained my composure, I motioned to the registered nurse to lean down in my direction. "Does uh, does uh, everyone here do that?" I whispered in her ear. "And by the way, what is he doing?"

She gave a little chuckle as she went back to filling out the baby's arm bands. "He's from Marin, honey."

That was it. That was the total explanation. Marin, I was soon to learn, is the county immediately north of the Golden Gate Bridge. I began to sense that maybe we weren't in Kansas anymore.

I witnessed another first-day cultural variation at the San Francisco General Hospital (SFGH) OB clinic. I stood in the hall outside one of the gazillion draped cubicles that mostly passed as exam rooms. All of the rooms were filled, largely with people for whom English was not even a second language.

As I dutifully waited for a nurse to accompany me in to examine the first patient, I noticed I was the only intern standing in the hall. A three-hundred-pound black nurse noticed the same thing and ambled over. Ah, I thought, She's going to lend assistance to the greenhorn.

"What you waitin' on, honey?"

"I was just waiting for a nurse, thank you."

"What fo, you needs somebody to hole yo hand?"

"Don't I need a chaperone in the room for an exam?"

Well, she looked at me like I was from not another state but a distant planet. "What you needs to do, doctor, is get yo happy ass in there and see the patient!"

"But . . ."

"The only butt I see out here is yo's, and iffin' yo wants to keep it outta the sling, yo best get in there now!"

Needless to say, the gentilities of the Old South were not recognized with your average Vietnamese patient in the San Francisco county hospital. I quickly entered the room only to realize that the person I really needed was the interpreter, who arrived in due time.

Now let's jump ahead about four weeks. It was midnight at Moffitt Hospital. Labor and delivery was on the fifteenth floor overlooking the old Kezar Stadium, Golden Gate Park, and, in the distance, the lights on the Golden Gate Bridge. I had had a month to adapt to a very different style of delivery, usually in a birthing room. While I was initially less adept, I had adjusted and, in fact, could at this point see considerable merit in unmedicated delivery in a nonsterile environment. As the midwives on staff taught me new tricks, I began to think I was pretty good at this and had seen the gamut of possible delivery styles.

My first educational experience that night came from a very attractive five-foot-ten Swedish blonde having her first child. She and her husband had spent early labor in one of the well-appointed birthing rooms, listening to music and mutually supporting each other with Lamaze technique. As it turned out, he was the Swedish consul to the United States in San Francisco.

When I went to check on her at about 1:00 a.m., she was in transition, or about eight centimeters dilated. This is usually the most painful part of a first labor, and I did not anticipate her delivery for at least several hours. Immediately after I told them this, she first opened the front of her gown, then shed it completely. Her husband helped her to a standing position next to the queen-sized bed.

# Disrobe Completely

I must have looked surprised because I remember her looking at me and asking if it was okay to be naked. Who was I to say no? She and her diplomat husband (who thankfully did not undress) proceeded to slow dance to Franz Schubert for the next two hours. It was actually remarkably beautiful. And definitely something I had not seen in Texas.

This couple taught me even more that night. After one and a half hours of pushing, during which she squatted and he supported her beneath the arms from behind, I delivered my first baby while lying flat on my back.

Not to be insensitive, but to imagine this, you have to have changed your own car's oil filter in the driveway. I might add that the anatomy of the pelvis is difficult to visualize normally, much less upside down and backwards. Pulling the delivering shoulder "down" beneath the pubic bone takes on a whole new complexity when you're in that position.

But we accomplished it together, and another beautiful little blonde, blue-eyed Swedish girl entered the world. The special nature of the moment of birth overcame any of my concerns about awkward positioning or unexpected nudity.

○○○

As I noted earlier, it was not only the mechanics of medicine I found markedly different in this new environment but the mechanics of life in a culture whose reputation for tolerance was known worldwide.

After only several days at SFGH, I was exposed to yet another novel situation for the novice physician. My chief resident told me to go work up an admission for a hysterectomy and bilateral oophorectomy (removal of ovaries) to be performed the following day. After clinic ended that evening around 7:00 p.m., I called the operator and was told that this patient was on ward 3D in bed 321B. It wasn't a GYN floor, but occasionally we had overflow to other wards, so I thought nothing of it. At the nurses' station I grabbed the chart with "Harrison" on it, and after a brief knock on the door, cruised into a room occupied only by a large, well-muscled, thick-bearded truck-driver type. I excused myself with a simple, "Sorry, wrong room," and didn't even wait for a response.

At the nurses' station, I asked an equally confused but slightly more annoyed clerk just where Miss Harrison had been deposited. She informed me that this was ward 3D. *Male* ward 3D. I mentioned to her that I was aware of that extremely useful fact, but was she aware that nevertheless, the computer felt 321B to be one Terry Harrison's room for the next several days? The clerk reached over the counter from her seated position, spun the chart around, and flipped open the plastic binder. Pointing to the stamp in the upper right corner of the first page, she looked at me and said, with her eyes only, "Whudduya think that says?"

Without further discussion, I picked up the phone and asked the operator to page my chief. In a few minutes she called back. "Say, Michelle, I'm on 3D looking for that woman you said needed the hyst tomorrow, and there don't seem to be any girl patients down here!"

"How do you know?" she responded.

"Excuse me?" I queried.

"Did you take a history or even introduce yourself?"

"Did I introduce myself as a gynecologist to a 250-pound guy with a beard? Well, no I didn't. Seemed like he might not like me interrupting his TV show."

"Well, *doctor* [too much emphasis on the second word here], maybe if you talk to Terry you'll learn to broaden your horizons and alter your expectations at the same time!"

"You're the boss."

With considerable trepidation, I reentered Terry's room. Needless to say, "HE" was not exactly the appropriate pronoun. Terry turned out to be a very pleasant transsexual. He had been taking male hormones for twenty years. While the sex-change operation from male to female is extremely well perfected, as I had witnessed in medical school, the female-to-male surgery is multistep and difficult, and at that time, led to extremely poor cosmetic results. Terry, as fate would have it, *was* in fact a long-distance trucker. Despite gainful employment, he had never acquired adequate funds for this uninsured procedure. So he led the life of a man, avoiding sexual encounters that might be disillusioning, to say the least, to new partners.

And he was hampered by one more little inconvenience. Heavy, extremely painful menstrual periods make long-distance trucking almost untenable for a woman; they make it even worse for a man. When Terry was in the company of others, he would explain the sudden onset of pains, the rushes to the bathroom, and the medications as the result of recurrent hernia pain.

The operation was a success. It was still remarkably strange, however, to be operating on female internal genitalia while at the same time being able to look over the drape and see the endotracheal tube protruding between a mustache and beard.

Some interesting discussions followed with regard to hormone replacement. While many women fear loss of estrogen function, this one positively rejoiced. We pointed out the benefits of estrogen replacement such as lower risk of heart attack, avoidance of hot flashes, avoidance of osteoporosis, etc. The patient pointed out that he felt one giant step closer to being in the body that he was wrongfully denied at birth by some undiscovered trick of hormonal biochemistry. No thanks, we could keep our estrogen replacement, and please, continue the testosterone injections during the recovery period.

Call me naive. I certainly was that. But I had begun to learn that we should treat all patients (read: people) with respect regardless of their outward appearance, just as we should regardless of their race.

○○○

# Not in Kansas Anymore

Now I'm basically a Southern boy, having been transplanted to Houston from New York while in the third grade. There are some things that a child of the South was just not adequately prepared for upon arrival in San Francisco. The stark natural beauty of every aspect of the Bay Area was one; the incredible chill of the ocean breeze coming off the Pacific even on what was ostensibly a warm summer day; and the beauty of Golden Gate Park. But even more startling at that point in my life was all the people of the same gender holding hands, kissing, lying on blankets, and just generally doing things that I had thought only people of the opposite gender did. Little did I know that some of the practices associated with what was then called an "alternative lifestyle" would meet up with me in the SFGH emergency room.

For example, the "gerbil problem" that's right, the furry little creatures that I had always mixed up with a guinea pig. Well, in San Francisco, at least in the early eighties, some of these furry little mammals met their end in a moderately grotesque fashion. While all humans have erogenous zones in and around their most posterior parts, apparently some of the men who lived in the Castro Valley district took this to a bit of an extreme. As any ER physician would gladly testify, a lot of different objects have been removed from the rectum. I myself had the pleasure of removing a wax candle stuck remarkably far inside of one my first patients in private practice. But in San Francisco, X-rays of the abdomen and pelvis revealed everything from sex toys made for this purpose to Coke bottles, candles, whip handles, staplers, soda cans, ping pong balls, golf balls, chess pieces, plastic baseball bats, garden hoses, kitchen utensils, rolling pins, bicycle pumps, racquet handles . . . the list is really longer than you need to hear.

However, the gerbil deal I have only witnessed in the SFGH emergency room and on multiple occasions, I might add. Evidently, forcing a live gerbil up the rectum followed by several more was a source of sexual excitation for some of the male community. The plan was that the little rodents would asphyxiate in the colon, and when they did so they would seize, and reportedly the sensation was, well, indescribable. That, I found quite credible. Part of my change of venue experience was working up a young man who had the misfortune to acquire a pair of gerbils who had managed to claw and chew their way through the wall of his transverse colon, spilling its contents into his peritoneal cavity in their death throws. As was clear from his KUB and upright abdominal X-ray, there was now free gas in the patient's abdominal cavity. He was in tremendous pain, febrile, and sweating like he lived in Dallas, not San Francisco. Because I was only an intern, I did not have the pleasure of witnessing the laparotomy and partial excision of his colon that subsequently saved his life.

I did, however, only two years later, get an opportunity to help a young man avoid a similar fate. I was paged at the usual 3:00 a.m., where incredibly, I was actually asleep in my call room, rare even for a third-year resident at the county. There was a garbled message in a foreign accent on the old radio pager to call my counterpart in general surgery. I dialed the number and was informed that a young man was about to have his abdomen opened and subsequently his colon in order to remove a hard, round object a little over two inches in diameter from the splenic flexure. The patient's partner informed us that the object seen on X-ray had been inserted in the rectum some six days previously with a cue stick. This, as it turns out, was completely appropriate, because the object in question was a pool ball. Specifically, it was the cue ball, but it unfortunately failed to reemerge from the same orifice into which they had inserted it so long ago. The patient had become extremely bloated and uncomfortable as of late, and when his condition began to include severe abdominal pain and protracted vomiting, the friend decided it was time for him to come in.

Now why, you might think to yourself, was I being paged? Well, just prior to the incision, an alert intern, of all people, queried the senior resident as to whether it might be possible to approach this problem in a different way. He apparently asked if there wasn't someone in the hospital who was actually *trained* to remove small, hard, round objects from body cavities.

I can promise you that when I arrived in the OR, armed with at least four different types of forceps, I had no idea if this was going to work. After looking at the X-rays and measuring the distance to the offending round ball usually employed for breaking and thus starting the game, I selected the long baby pipers. This forcep is normally used for the after-coming head of a breech. (Today, of course, we use the ole Bard-Parker for the breech—the brand name of knife used when doing a cesarean.) The piper is oddly shaped with long, curving stems and a set of small, cupped, curved blades at the end. I saw no way I could possibly get to the cue ball, much less open the blades wide enough to get around it if I ever got there.

"Tell me about the colon. I'm more of a vagina guy, if you know what I mean. How far can I open this thing?" I looked over my mask at the senior surgery resident standing by the OR table, arms folded, and I believe smirking, beneath his mask.

"Not sure, my friend. Pretty far I would think. Wasn't it you who helped me last month on that girl who got raped with a city fire-hose nozzle? You remember, the one with the ruptured vaginal vault, ruptured anus, ruptured rectum, ruptured colon, torn kidney, ruptured spleen?"

Yeah, I remembered. And yes, unfortunately, that had been me who first saw the seventeen-year-old girl in the trauma room of the ER and then was in and out of her thirteen-hour-long surgery. She died in the ICU. Her attacker was still at large.

"Yeah, that was me . . . I get your point." The patient was completely asleep, and we had an ultrasound tech present to help us "approach" the problem, as it were. Remarkably, after about twenty minutes of struggling, a whole lot of lubricant, and some deft maneuvering, we delivered a bouncing, healthy, baby cue ball! We were all pretty pleased with ourselves, having avoided an exploratory laparotomy, but I think the pathologist was less than amused when we sent the ball to the lab in a bucket of formalin and gave it initial Apgar scores of zero and zero.

○○○

San Francisco was indeed a change of venue. From the different medical instruments and techniques to a culture with totally different customs and new definitions of the norm, it brought a shift of reference points far beyond what I had expected. But physicians are trained to adapt to new situations. If you can't adapt, you can't very well deal with that surgical problem that crops up without warning when you least expect it (not to mention *where* you least expect it).

# A Radical Concept

*Ask the children of a physician where Dad (or Mom, as the case may be) was during their first dance recital or their first T-ball game or their sixteenth birthday party. "The hospital" will likely be the answer, because the only other possible response would be "asleep."*

*Call it drive, call it dedication, call it foolish, call it anything you want, but it's a fact: physicians learn to subjugate the wants and needs of their families and friends and even themselves to those of their patients, who soon become the priority. The doctor may be due at home for dinner. The doctor may be a walking zombie after thirty-six hours without sleep. But diagnostic tests, IV placements, wound changes, record keeping, and family conferences must go on. Even before my children could tell time, they learned from their mother that "on time" didn't apply to Dad. If I swore I'd be home at 6:00 p.m., it might well be 9:00 p.m., and that meant after bedtime—another twenty-four hours without seeing Papa.*

Sleep. Now there is a completely radical concept! If you want to get any physician in a surgical subspecialty excited to the point where he makes your one-year-old, non-neutered Labrador surrounded by bitches in heat look tame by comparison, offer him three hours of uninterrupted sleep.

I do not exaggerate. I know from personal experience that the average intern/resident—despite days, weeks, or months of abstinence—can fall asleep while an attractive, libidinous, naked member of the opposite sex lies beside him.

This is no reflection on said physician's degree of interest in the act of coitus or other related modes of sexual interaction. It merely shows he's got his priorities in order. Those of us who have spent years running up sleep deficits that make Washington's deficits look like pocket change know that an opportunity to hit the pillow is not to be taken lightly.

Sleep. Ah, sleep. Sleep is not just a steak cooked to perfection. Sleep is not just that feeling of taking your ski boots off after six hours on the slopes. Sleep is not just removing your hard contacts after thirty-six hours of wear. Sleep is not even that muscle convulsing, warm, wet waves of intense pleasure that accompanies the temporary insanity of orgasm.

No. Sleep is better! Much, much better!

When I was in college, my older brother (now a heart surgeon) used to tell me that he fell asleep in the elevators. I scoffed, not being naive enough to believe his tales of woe. Right, I thought. And weren't you the one who had to trudge twelve miles to school in the snow with sixty pounds of books on your back because they didn't invent the school bus until three years later when I started kindergarten? Of course, it turns out that I was the little brother of little faith. When my turn to sleep by necessity in odd places finally arrived, it proved more dangerous to the public than sleeping in elevators.

Now keep in mind that sleep deprivation is probably the most effective form of torture used in covert intelligence gathering throughout the world. Amnesty International has it listed in its official menu of things civilized governments don't do to people. We don't really know what sleep is, what it does, how it does it, or much about it at all, except that a certain amount of it is absolutely necessary for proper cognition, orientation, memory, as well as all other identifiable emotional and physical functioning. Deprived of sleep long enough, you first become lethargic, then disoriented, then agitated and then quite frankly, stark, raving mad. Then you go see the patient in 321B.

The elevator nap, a.k.a. Dover dozing, is really a safety mechanism. If it weren't for these quick encounters with the sandman, many of the nation's people would be under the knife of agitated, disoriented, just short of Looney-Tunes surgeons.

I have seen colleagues fall asleep while eating, engaged in public speaking, riding in elevators, riding in ambulances, driving their cars, holding retractors, taking objective tests, reading X-rays, presenting a case to their pimper (see "The Strong Survive"), riding a bike, playing tennis, performing a pelvic exam, or listening to a patient's chest.

The remarkable thing is that I have yet to witness a major error that I felt was caused by sleep deprivation in the treatment of a patient. There is truly something remarkable about the old adrenal glands. If a patient is in deep *kemshee* (doo-doo), you can pull out all the stops instantly, awaken from a dead stupor, and—on *very* little sleep—do exactly what you were trained to do.

I'm sure the lay public views this phenomenon as less than safe. Some states have naively instituted legislation to limit the number of hours in a shift for medical personnel in training at state-funded institutions. Ha! Who are they kidding? At SFGH, when you've been up for the last thirty-eight hours but still have twenty-six patients to round on, one crisis working in the ER, another disaster in ICU, and my replacement just as bombed in the operating room, what are you supposed to do? Saunter over to the time clock and punch out? You work until the work is done and you're covered by the next schmuck. Period. End of story. Rules changes since 2001 have limited shifts within some residencies, but the simple fact is the rules become more like guidelines when a warm body is needed and the team is overwhelmed.

Let the legislators mosey on over to their nearest teaching hospital and take a look at who's delivering the care. Let them find a way to triple the MDs in county facilities nationwide (hello, tax hikes), and then talk to us about twelve-hour shifts and getting adequate sleep. When you're bleeding to death from the bullet in your chest, a sleepy chest cutter is better than no chest cutter, right?

Now, admittedly there's a lighter side to this issue. Every spouse of an intern can tell you of the lovely, romantic anniversary dinner that was spoon-fed to the barely conscious intern propped up on the couch. Said meal lasted only until said intern could be sleepwalked to the bedroom for the usual six-hour respite before the thirty-six-hour cycle began again.

I would literally awaken to the 5:30 a.m. alarm and have no memory of how I got home from the hospital, ate dinner, took off my clothes, and fell into bed. I couldn't begin to tell you the number of nights I wandered for blocks in the San Francisco fog, having no idea where I'd parked my Celica with its 180,000 miles in the early morning of the day before.

But patients may rest assured, the danger only began when I got behind the wheel. If you have a patient's belly open and she's bleeding to death from a ruptured ectopic pregnancy, it doesn't matter when you slept last; baby, you are *wide awake*. But when you're in the familiar comfort of your driver's seat, essentially guiding the car on autopilot through the same streets, the same turns, the same hills, the same lights, you can drift a bit.

Take the time I woke up with the bumper of my Celica on the trailer hitch of the pickup in front of me. Take the time I rolled backwards down one of those world-renowned San Francisco hills in my week-old Jeep Cherokee and smashed into a nurse's day-old Mazda RX-7, completely filleting the hood from latch to windshield. Take the time the trolley-car conductor had to shake me awake while my car straddled the rails, detaining angry tourists from their intended spending sprees. Take the time I drove the wrong way down the one-way street in Golden Gate Park, stopping only nose-to-nose with one of those funny cars with the flashing lights on top. Keep in mind, these are only some of my exploits. During any twenty-four-hour period, a big-city public-hospital may send 100 to 150 sleep-deprived interns and hundreds of slightly less sleep-deprived residents out on the highways. Besides those "Quiet" signs that surround hospitals, maybe we need "Caution: Interns Dozing!" signs as well.

After two years in San Francisco, my wife wanted more room than the eight-hundred-square-foot walk-up that we shared with our Siamese. I said, "Why on earth would you want to move? We just got here."

That's when, using her laptop computer, my wife pointed out that I had in fact actually "lived" in the apartment five-fold less time than she had or the equivalent of four and one half months. No wonder I felt like we'd just arrived. We further calculated that I spent 90% of my time in that apartment unconscious, so that I only remembered being there the equivalent of thirteen and one-half days! It was a moot point anyway. On $13,000 a year in the most expensive city in America, Russian Hill wasn't exactly beckoning.

So sleep. Enjoy it. Revel in it. Wrap it around you like a down comforter in winter; splash in it like a cool running stream in summer. But don't ever take it for granted. I guarantee your doctor doesn't.

# Good Grief

*It comes in many forms, grief. It can be a silence, a contemplation of something once possessed but lost long ago. Or it can be more immediate. Then it comes in waves, rolling, relentless, inescapable. It can be so oppressive that it actually takes on physical qualities. Thick, seemingly impenetrable, sometimes even suffocating.*

*Everyone has things to mourn in their lives. We all grieve on the passing of loved ones. But the commonality lays only with expected deaths. Most people expect their grandparents to die before their parents and their parents before their siblings or spouses and themselves before their children.*

*Physicians, in company only with the clergy and the undertaker, must deal not only with these deaths but also with those most horrible events for which the patient and her loved ones are completely unprepared. The most stressful event that a human can experience is roundly agreed to be the loss of a child. It appears to matter little whether that child is a minute old or seventy years old. The twenty-year-old mother of the term stillbirth may well understand the anguish of the ninety-year-old who has outlived her seventy-year-old son.*

*It was at San Francisco General where I first witnessed the inconsolable sadness that comes from such a loss—and tasted the bitter dregs of abject failure as a doctor.*

# Good Grief

The young woman was eighteen, an indigenous Laotian who presented with no prenatal care at thirty-four-weeks gestation but nevertheless had her extended family with her. She had become sick several days before with vomiting, jaundice, diarrhea, progressive fatigue and disorientation, and, finally, incoherence. It was only then that her family rejected provincial attempts at therapy and called an ambulance.

Shortly after the young woman's arrival in the labor and delivery department, a sonogram revealed that the fetus had not survived the rapid onset of her mother's undiagnosed and untreated toxemia. The disease process had left the mother horribly swollen, hypertensive, close to coma, and with rapidly deteriorating liver and kidney function. She was, however, in labor at eight centimeters and would deliver soon.

Largely through hand gestures, we let the family know the fetus had died. As for the girl, the only Lao interpreters on staff were not of her Mien mountain area and knew little of her dialect. So, minutes after her arrival, knowing nothing of her infant's fate, she began bearing down visibly with the strain of impending delivery recognizable worldwide. She was rushed on a gurney to a delivery/OR and placed on the table in stirrups.

At that time, the families were not allowed in the delivery rooms, and I remember the nurses and the interpreter physically restraining the woman's young husband and distraught parents. From where I sat at the foot of the table I could see them sobbing and shouting intermittently through the glass wall that divided the OR from the rest of labor and delivery proper.

The pain of the delivery had momentarily brought the girl to full consciousness, and she struggled against the anesthesiologist's attempts to mask her with some nitrous oxide. Despite her inability to understand us or cooperate, the delivery itself was uncomplicated. When she saw her bloated, meconium (dark green)-stained, lifeless child, she began to roll her head back and forth and moan in an indescribable wail.

# Disrobe Completely

I sewed her perineum rapidly and was just about finished when the anesthesiologist noted a further loss of orientation and a froth bubbling from her mouth. Within seconds the patient's wailing was replaced by a sickening gurgle, then stillness. We called a code at that point and immediately began CPR while the anesthesiologist placed the endotracheal tube. I'll never forget the fluid that jetted out of that tube with each and every chest compression. She literally drowned in her own secretions as the capillaries of her lungs gave in to the effects of the unseen amniotic fluid embolus that was robbing her of life beneath our hands and high-tech instruments.

She began to bleed vaginally, gushing like a bathtub faucet. When a bolus of amniotic fluid enters the veins in the wall of the uterus, it can travel to the lungs through the right heart. There, it blocks oxygen exchange and essentially suffocates the patient. The onset of bleeding was due to an over-tired uterus unable to contract combined with abnormalities of blood clotting that accompany severe toxemia or preeclampsia. During the next two hours, with at least twelve team members in the room, she received over thirty units of blood, twenty liters of saline, and sixty units of fresh, frozen plasma and was cardioverted (shocked) five times. Yet nothing could halt the inexorable approach of doom set in motion by this rare embolic process. When we finally called a stop to it, we were literally ankle-deep in body fluids.

By the time she was declared dead, a Mien Laotian sanitation worker had been summoned from his home in Portrero Hill to act as interpreter. At first, the family simply could not believe that their loved one was gone. After steadfastly refusing to accept our account of her death, they insisted on seeing her before transfer to the morgue. She was still in that God-awful room with her blood on the floor and the endotracheal tube in her mouth, further distorting the features already altered by bloating and discoloration. I shall never forget her father sinking to his knees, rolling on the floor, and beating the blood-soaked linoleum with both fists clenched. His moan sounded exactly the same as the one his daughter had delivered hours before at first sight of her dead child. Nearly everyone in the room was crying.

All of us interns and junior residents learned a lot in the ensuing five days as the case was researched and presented at conference. We learned, when the labs came back, of her preeclampsia (toxemia), the ensuing abruption (placental separation), the fetal death, and the coagulation abnormalities brought on by that process, combined with the prolonged retained dead fetus, combined with liver failure, combined with the crowning blow of amniotic fluid embolus. But those of us that were there learned much more than the physiology.

Those of us who had never faced the death of a patient in our care will not forget that day. Mortality comes crashing home when you see the life of a teenager pumped out onto the floor.

I heard a message in the common moan of husband and daughter, a message that shaped me as a physician far more than the understanding of her disease process. This message has many layers, but certainly a central part of it is that what we do is very important to people. Oh, they may not say it much anymore, but people really do put their lives in doctors' hands, and the loss of any life brings home the gravity of our responsibility. I think all physicians get that portion of the message.

There is another part of the message that most, but not all, physicians come to understand: our patients expect more than medical expertise and judgment. They expect us to be healers of both body and spirit. And yet, too great an emotional investment in the spiritual renewal of a devastated patient or loved one can rapidly destroy a practicing physician.

It is the tightrope between callous aloofness on the one side and complete surrender to despair on the other that the physician must walk. In recent months, I or one of my partners had to tell a twenty-seven-year-old just back from her honeymoon that she had breast cancer; remove the cancerous kidney of a woman twenty-eight-weeks pregnant with twins who thought she would never live to see their second birthdays; console the mother of an eight-week-old girl who died of SIDS; help the mother of a two-year-old crushed beneath a garage door operated by her five-year-old brother; comfort the mother of a two-year-old who pulled over his dresser drawers and suffocated himself; support a thirty-seven-year-old woman just after discovering on ultrasound that after eight years of infertility and subsequent successful in vitro fertilization, her twelve-week fetus was dead; and meet repeatedly with parents whose baby had died moments after birth of meconium aspiration, while the grandparents and great-grandparents looked on in the birthing room.

In early 2006, I had to sit down with a patient of mine of twenty years, who now at forty-four years old, had received the independent diagnoses of Hodgkin's lymphoma and breast cancer within three weeks of each other! She had three teenagers and a husband to care for.

Such events, while rare in the lives of most people, are almost daily occurrences for the physician. Many physicians become emotionally involved in the care of their patients, and rightly so. Many times I have cried with a patient or their family because I truly shared in their anguish. Certainly there are those trained specifically in dealing with grief—psychologists, social workers, and chaplains. But the family physician of long standing can help, perhaps more than anyone else, with healthy grief counseling.

But who will heal the healer? There is always the next patient, and that patient also wants and deserves the doctor's emotional investment. Moments after discussing the probability of ovarian cancer with a woman who has just seen her own mass on the ultrasound screen, the doctor must walk into the next room and share the joy of the long-term infertility patient who sees her tiny fetus on that same screen for the very first time.

It takes tremendous energy to alter one's demeanor rapidly and repeatedly, day in and day out, changing your mood to mirror the patient's. A few physicians cope by withdrawing emotionally. So far that hasn't happened to me, and I hope it never does. Feeling too much may mean a slight loss of objectivity, but the human interaction fostered by empathy outweighs any inefficiency.

When my son was four years old, he came into my bedroom one of the afternoons I had off. I had just finished talking to my minister about the death of a newborn. Although I knew I was not responsible, I was distraught over the grief and anger of the patient's family. I had been sobbing to the extent that when Andy saw my face, he started crying too. Later, he told his teacher at my wife's Bible study fellowship that his daddy had cried because a baby had died. He was told that it was good his daddy could cry over things like that, and Andy seemed satisfied.

Well, overall, I think the teacher was correct. It is good that a physician can cry like that. But it didn't feel good—not at all.

So the next time a physician strikes you as cold or unfeeling, think about what he might have had to tell the patient right before you. Some of us just shift gears a little faster than others. We only hope that rapid gear shifts won't leave the mechanism stripped or worse, replaced with a "managed care automatic transmission," whereby the doctor makes a cash transaction with the "customer," and the patient ceases to exist.

The degree to which the doctor can truly participate in the spiritual healing of his patient cannot help but be linked to the longevity of their relationship. The doctor-patient relationship is indeed defined by the revelation of intimacies, the counseling through difficult times, and the gradual relaxation of defenses between two people that occurs with the development of trust. As we shall see, the health care provider (with whom you have spoken only once) at your health-maintenance organization may not be able to deal with whatever grief you might face in quite the same manner as your personal physician could have.

# Disrobe Completely

I wrote this chapter in the evening of a particularly harrowing day. After four days out of town, I returned to find that one of my long-term infertility patients had lost her pregnancy at twenty-two weeks due to an unexpected rupture of membranes and ensuing infection and labor. My partners had done all the right things. They had behaved professionally and compassionately. They had explained everything to the best of their ability. Still, this morning, the day after her loss for which I was not present, she burst into tears and held open her arms when I walked into her room.

I sat on her bed and held her in my arms for several moments until her sobs subsided. Her husband had his hand on my shoulder throughout and didn't hide his own tears. Despite a packed schedule, I spent the next forty-five minutes talking with the two of them. We covered ground I knew my partners had already covered, but they wanted to hear it from me. We discussed the emotions she would experience, from denial to anger to bewilderment to fear, and finally to resolution. We talked about the future. We talked about whatever needed talking about. Despite the guilt I always feel at not being there for the patient when a crisis occurs, she said as I left, "Thank you for being here. You don't know what a difference it makes."

I do know what a difference it makes, to me and to the patient. I know that without the ability to touch a patient and relieve her suffering there would be no reason to do what I do for a living. And even though there may be many doctors who don't take advantage of these windows of opportunity to truly heal, many of us do. I don't want you to lose the opportunity to have a doctor who really knows and cares for you, instead of a doctor who has only seen you once or has never seen you at all and who, after all, gets off at five o'clock sharp every day.

# Let 'Em See You Sweat

*Doctors are in no way infallible. In fact, our mistakes may be more evident than those of most professionals due to the nature of our work. If, in a frenzied moment, the doctor makes a flawed judgment, the good doctor recognizes the errors, makes appropriate changes, and moves on.*

*But you can't learn from mistakes if you won't acknowledge them. The patient must view the doctor as even-keeled, as William Osler counseled, but the med-school admonition to "never let them see you sweat" is bad advice for the doctor-patient relationship. A patient cannot trust a physician who perceives himself as infallible, because inevitably the doctor will prove he is not—perhaps at the patient's expense.*

In *Kindergarten Cop*, the harried Arnold Schwarzenegger gets a splitting headache from dealing with his pint-sized charges. When his partner offers her own diagnosis and insists that the pain might have a more ominous origin, Arnold lays down the law, "EETS NOTTA TOOMAH!"

No book focusing on the making of a surgeon (that is, gynecologic) could fail to include the well-meaning misdiagnoses made by nongynecologists when it comes to the female reproductive organs. Let's look first at the "It's not a tumor!" category.

I was awakened one night at around 3:30 a.m. (yet again) while on call as a junior resident at San Francisco General Hospital (SFGH). This was unusual only in that I was actually asleep and miraculously had been for over forty-five minutes. The three interns covering labor and delivery and the ER were evidently in total control or, alternatively, had nothing to do.

In any event, the page was from a senior internal-medicine resident who was screening intern presentations in the ER. He listened to the case of a Vietnamese woman who was writhing in pain, had her hands clutched to her abdomen, and evidently had a large pelvic-abdominal tumor. As is often the case with indigenous, non-English-speaking Asian patients, she evidently had not recently been a supplicant at this particular shrine of Western medicine. It's not uncommon for such patients to arrive in the emergency room with advanced malignancies in a crisis stage.

The internal-medicine resident, being the diligent fellow that he was, had personally examined the patient and confirmed the intern's findings. There was a large, rock-hard, pelvic mass at the apex of the vagina, which seemed to extend in an irregular configuration all the way to the sternum. There was a small amount of blood from the opening of the cervix on speculum exam, but the upper vagina otherwise looked normal to visual inspection.

When I arrived in the tiny curtained space in the packed emergency ward, I discovered what can only be described as bedlam. The patient, who appeared to be about seventeen years old, was sweating heavily, flushed, and agitated. There was a woman by the head of the bed in tears, with her arms and upper body thrown across the thrashing patient's chest. Furthermore, the tiny space contained the resident, the emergency room intern, a nurse, and the two security men restraining the patient's father, who was babbling unintelligibly and gesticulating wildly with alternating arms, as he yanked away each arm in turn from those trying to restrain him. He seemed to be hurling most of his Vietnamese invective at our hapless internal-medicine resident. In this quiet, calm group of professionals, they needed me?

Anybody appraising this situation could tell one thing immediately: there were just too many people screaming in this tiny space. I asked security to remove the distraught gentleman and requested that the two other physicians give me a moment alone with the patient. When the noise level was down to only the patient's groans and the mother's sobs, I asked one of the only things I know how to say in French, "When was your last period?"

Well, the question seemed to silence the mother. The teenager looked up and said, "I don't know," which was about the only other thing I know in French. With the nurse's help, the patient allowed a brief bimanual pelvic exam to confirm the impending birth. Quite remarkably, after we communicated this upcoming event with some unmistakable international sign language, the mother began once again to sob and wail and the daughter to thrash and groan.

The other physicians were, of course, mortified at my findings, almost to the point of self-vaporization. Once a translator had been obtained, however, it became clear that only the patient herself secretly suspected her actual diagnosis. The parents practiced the Eastern version of Western denial, believing steadfastly that this occurrence was not possible since their daughter had not yet enjoyed sexual congress. I was tempted to tell the translator that she may not have enjoyed it, but she'd definitely had it. I remembered my professional code of conduct at the last instant.

This is not as outrageous as it seems. Doctors are no more omniscient than they are infallible, and many a patient has intentionally or inadvertently misled those attempting to care for her. In this case, denial was so manifest that this Vietnamese family either really didn't know what was happening or considered it so unlikely that they denied the logical findings of their own senses. Thanks to their demeanor on arrival and thereafter, the intern was sucked in completely.

And who can blame him? All doctors have seen people with large, previously undiagnosed cancers. The family's agitation told the unfortunate intern that something extremely grave must be happening here, making it easy for him to overlook the patient's youth, the fact that her pain came in waves, and even that on exam this mass felt just like a baby was supposed to feel. The resident, listening to hundreds of case presentations that evening, had hurried his exam and simply bought what the intern had told him.

Now, before you think that I'm libeling another specialty, scope out the following scenario. Two years before I came to SFGH, there was a case that will live in infamy, a case that the responsible doctor will carry like a millstone around his neck forever.

Once again, it is 3:00 a.m., a favorite time for disasters in medicine. The chief OB resident is called to the ER for a screaming, morbidly obese woman who is bleeding vaginally and clutching her generous abdomen.

"The baby! The baby!" she shrieked. "Oh my God! My God! The baby's coming RIGHT NOW!"

Well, that kind of talk is bound to get attention. The nurses had listened for fetal heart tones and reported them as 70 (normal 120-160). Without immediate intervention, the fetus might die or be severely damaged. The senior resident had to make the decision as the patient was rushed on a gurney to L&D. He was waiting to examine her when she was wheeled in from the elevator. His bimanual exam revealed a single footling breech, and the patient was taken around the corner to the OR where she was crashed (put rapidly to sleep) and sliced open vertically for a STAT cesarean section.

Everything went well with the surgery, despite the patient's massive size. She made a very nice recovery. The only little hang-up was that she hadn't been pregnant—ever.

Well, how is this possible? you ask. Were these doctors just careless or complete idiots? Ask an attorney. They were negligent, weren't they? The answer, of course, is that they were none of these. They were human. Patient's heart is pounding—so is yours. Patient's afraid her baby's going to die—so are you.

The woman was not really pregnant. She was, however, quite sick. She suffered from pseudocyesis, a very real psychiatric diagnosis in which a schizophrenic patient, very convincingly I might add, believes herself to be pregnant. The disorder presumably derives from a fervent desire to have a child in the face of some reason why this cannot be the case at the time—sterility, no sex partner, etc.

The senior resident, not unlike our intern in the ER, not unlike the nurse who heard the patient's pulse and believed it to be a fetus's heart, was completely sucked in. He *knew* this lady was pregnant before he examined her. Thus, the tampon he felt during the pelvic exam quite naturally became a foot prolapsing through the cervix.

The patient, incidentally, was not angry in the least. She did, however, grieve the loss of her imaginary child, and only when she was admitted to the psych ward on the first floor was it discovered that she had been discharged one week before. Diagnosis? You guessed it! Pseudocyesis.

Maybe this debacle was a failing on the part of all the people that cared for her. Maybe it was only a failing on the part of a choked medical records system. But it certainly demonstrates the fact that physicians and nurses are human and empathize with patients whether they want to or not. And it reminds us that separating rational thought from adrenaline-driven impulses is difficult to do.

○○○

All physicians have found themselves in situations where letting the patient see you sweat, while uncomfortable, was better for all concerned. Virtually all medical organizations and colleges have recently changed their recommendations for how physicians should behave in their relationship to patients and families in difficult circumstances. Specifically in the difficult situation when we realize that we've made a mistake. The unwritten code for the most recent litigious decades has been the same across specialties and across the nation. If you made a mistake, keep cool and don't volunteer anything. Explain things if necessary in terms of complications, but avoid intimating that the outcome was in any way tied to an error on your part. Much of this attitude was fostered by our malpractice carriers whose lawyers truly believed that "anything you say now can and will be used against you in a court of law."

Many physicians, for many years, have been extremely uncomfortable with this perspective. Those of us who care for people for a living desperately want the freedom to be honest with them. And yes, sometimes the things to which we confess might be used against us later, but more often they are not. Why? Because patients want an honest relationship as well, and they appreciate our candor when it is called for.

I hadn't been in private practice for too many years when I had the opportunity to operate on a young woman for endometriosis that was thought to be contributing to her several years of infertility. Her name was Mariah and as fate would have it, her father was one of my former clinical professors in Houston who had achieved a modicum of notoriety with a clinical invention related to preventing second-trimester pregnancy loss. Well, if you're under thirty like I was at the time, you might as well have one of your oral examiners under the knife as have the daughter of a former Ob/Gyn professor! Talk about "let 'em see you sweat." To add insult to injury (no pun intended), her brother-in-law was a well-known personal injury attorney in town! No pressure!

Well, she was a slender, pretty girl, and her laparoscopy went without a hitch. She was operated on in a surgery center adjacent to the hospital, recovered for several hours, and was sent home from there. When I had introduced the laparoscope (a telescope inserted through the navel to observe and/or operate within the pelvis and abdomen), I saw minimal amounts of endometriosis displayed on the TV screen. Using a KTP laser, popular at the time, I vaporized the small amount of disease present, chromotubated (flushed dye through her fallopian tubes to prove they were open), took pictures, and then removed the abdominal instruments and sewed the two small incisions closed. The nurses removed the speculum and uterine manipulator from the vagina, as well as the Foley catheter from the bladder, and the patient went to the recovery room without incident.

On Monday morning, my partner John, who had been on call the night before, called me and asked if I remembered anything strange about Mariah's case? No, I told him; everything went off without a hitch. "Well," he said, "she called me about midnight and reported that she had gone to use the restroom and something metal had clanked into the toilet!"

"You have *got* to be kidding me!" Unfortunately, though John is a joker, he was not joking this time.

"She said at first when she called her husband into the bathroom and showed him the piece of metal, he was positive it was a part of the toilet."

"What on earth?"

"Listen, listen. I reassured them at the time. She was in no pain and not bleeding, so I asked them to bring the metal piece in on Saturday morning."

"This cannot be happening! Do you know who she is? She's the daughter of one of my old professors at Baylor and the sister-in-law of the plaintiff's attorney by the same name!"

"Oops."

"Yeah, oops is right."

"Well, you might want to give them a call. They did bring it in the next day, and it was the steel acorn off the end of the Cohen's cannula."

"Oh my God, you cannot be serious! The circulating nurse took out the Cohen's while I was sewing up her belly. Do you think it came unscrewed and she just didn't notice the tip was missing?"

"That's all I can think of. Look, no harm, no foul. There was no damage done. But yeah, you better give them a call."

Okay, if you looked up the term "sheepish" in the dictionary in around 1986, there was a full-color picture of me in the margin. I called Mariah, did a full *mea culpa*, and basically was as effusively apologetic as I could be. She was nicer than could be expected, but then I had to call and talk to her father. I don't even remember that conversation. I think I may have totally blanked it out . . . or maybe I fainted during it.

What I do know is that Mariah got pregnant the following cycle, and I was released from the proverbial doghouse just as quickly as I had been thrown into it. I now have pictures of her three kids above my credenza and a crystal clock she gave me after she found out she was pregnant. I suppose this was one of those situations where there was no such thing as plausible deniability, but still, being as open as possible with an error, harmless or not, is critical to the doctor-patient relationship.

It was the startling recommendation in 2001 from the American College of Obstetrics and Gynecology and the American Medical Society as well as the medical-legal community that we—are you ready for this—*apologize* as soon as possible after an unexpected outcome or clear-cut error. It is becoming official that it is okay to do what all of us have always wanted to do from the start but that the attorneys have always said was tantamount to professional and legal suicide. Chalk one up for medical ethics. Official approval for honesty and contrition. Gotta love that! Now you *can* let 'em see you sweat, the ability to do so having always been a critical character trait in my estimation.

ooo

Ten years ago, I had the privilege of being an observer in a sophisticated Boeing 767 virtual-reality simulator. Practicing takeoff from O'Hare into a thunderstorm with downbursts, both of the experienced pilots killed us three times apiece. Even knowing what to expect, they made the same instinctive error repeatedly. Why? Because they were forced to react quickly without opportunity for contemplation. Even in a simulator, you could feel their fear like a palpable thing. In slow motion, they would have realized that forcing the nose up while averting an aborted takeoff, nevertheless crashed the tail section into the runway and destroyed the aircraft. The flight computer in the same situation never erred on multiple trials, but the flight computer knows nothing about fear.

We can all be led astray by our initial impressions and be further confused by the emotions of those around us. Learning to evaluate "just the facts, ma'am" is difficult but essential for all of us, whether doctor, lawyer, pilot, or Indian chief, if we want to make the right decisions. Don't get me wrong. There are many instances where the pilot can outperform the computer by virtue of his human qualities of judgment, perseverance, and experience. By the same token, as pointed out previously, the doctor who can empathize may better serve some patient needs by demonstrating his compassion and thus his humanity.

Being a good doctor requires the cool, clockwork rationality of the flight computer—and more. While the pilot must recognize his own emotions and fears but never show them to the crew or passengers, the doctor must learn that his own emotions and fears are the same as his patients' and that occasionally revealing them can be beneficial to the doctor-patient relationship. Achieving the desired outcome while still remaining human requires both compassion and self-discipline. These virtues are learned not in the flight simulator of medical school but in the cockpit, in the air, in real practice with precious lives in your care. Every now and then, let 'em see you sweat. They won't trust you completely if you don't.

# Big Sucker, Idn'it?

---

*"Walk a mile in my shoes." Or just walk to the bathroom dragging an IV and wondering if your behind is showing through that ridiculous hospital gown designed by La Voyeur. We doctors can intellectually acknowledge the fear, the uncertainty, the embarrassment, and most of all the helplessness of our patients, but being patients ourselves changes mere sympathy to empathy. Once we've been "the broken leg in 135" or "the gall bladder in 316," we cannot help but meet the next patient's needs better than we did before our own health crisis.*

---

I had awakened a decade ago with what I thought was the usual morning stiffness—a gift, as we all know, from the God of Approaching Forty. I intended to head for the shower, first making the obligatory stop at my top bureau drawer for the morning's 800 mg of ibuprofen. Unfortunately, as I attempted to stand beside the bed, an excruciating pain shot down the back of my left leg to my heel.

As if that weren't bad enough, my foot suddenly began ignoring the important messages being sent earthward by areas of higher brain function. I had to drag it behind me, the perfect picture of the classic "foot drop" and a virtual tribute to Charles Laughton in *The Hunchback of Notre Dame*. Sitting, lying, or squatting brought no relief to the intensifying sciatica.

I had previously experienced the complete paralysis of paraspinous muscle spasm, spending two scenic days in traction on the orthopedic floor at my very own hospital. On this occasion, however, the muscle spasm was mercifully absent. Consequently, I was able to drive to work after a fashion, lying on my left side with the seat reclined, working both pedals with my good right foot. The pain down my buttock, thigh, and calf was excruciating. Phenomenally, I killed no one on the drive to the hospital.

Using all my worldly influence as a frequent and loyal referring physician, I was able to finagle a visit with the neurosurgeon—*two days* later. They might as well have told me they'd slip me in when the House of Representatives has a Republican majority!* Martyr that I am, I literally dragged myself through the next forty-eight hours, seeing patients but canceling surgery left and right, and, of course, complaining bitterly every gimpy step of the way.

On the appointed day, I spent the better part of the afternoon at the Southwest Imaging Center, a large facility that takes up the bottom two floors of one of the professional buildings on the hospital campus. When I arrived at the window wearing scrubs and a white coat, I was strafed with the silent appraisal of the waiting room's septuagenarian and octogenarian occupants. There were no vacant seats, but this wasn't all bad since sitting was excruciating. I leaned against a column and tried to concentrate on a copy of *Preventive Health*, one of my personal favorites.

After less than three minutes a technician called out, "Dr. Thurston?" If looks could really kill, I would have been vaporized in an instant. Fifteen pairs of tired but intense eyes set in careworn faces bored through my head with laser-like intensity. I felt like an ax murderer just released on a technicality. (Thankfully, as it turned out, I wasn't receiving special treatment. The technician told me that none of the other patients were waiting for the MRI machine.)

The technician turned me over to a late-fiftyish schoolmarm of a nurse who directed me to a small changing room and instructed me to disrobe completely, put on the gown, sit on the bench outside the change room, and wait.

*Archaeological evidence that this phrase was written before Nov 8, 1994*

# Disrobe Completely

I pulled the curtain, undressed, and fretted momentarily about where to leave my wallet. Finally, I just put it in my front pants pocket with the keys, somehow reassured that no thief would ever look further than the right hip pocket for a wallet. (The same rationale that operates when you "hide" your wallet in your tennis shoe while you swim in the ocean.)

As I donned the threadbare hospital gown, open to the rear, I made the executive decision that "completely" didn't mean removing my underwear. Feeling ridiculous, I threw open the curtain and prepared to lurch the short distance to the bench. A half-glass door immediately across the hallway opened and, with no schoolmarm in sight, out swept Penelope Cruz in a nurse's uniform, a very tight, curve-hugging nurse's uniform. She tossed her perfect, wavy brunette locks over her shoulder in that provocative way that little girls must learn to do in kindergarten. Her smile-giggle revealed a million jiggawatts of perfect pearly whites.

"Everything, doctor. You'll need to take off everything, including your underwear. You're up, so I'll wait here for you." She shooed me back to the curtained cloister, arms out straight, hands bent down at the wrist, fingers flicking back and forth. My God, it was Marilyn Monroe in *The Seven Year Itch*!

I retreated to the changing room and, for no earthly reason, found that I regretted my dark socks, moderate pot belly, and love handles. I was reasonably happy in my marriage. Why should I care what Marilyn or Penelope or whoever thinks about my socks? Right. What if she puts me on the table, and I get . . . you know, get a . . . Why the good Lord made Mr. Happy function completely independently of the conscious male mind is beyond me. It is also a corollary to this axiom that the harder one tries to avoid, well, tenting one's gown, the more likely it becomes. Despite the almost unimaginable shooting pain in my left cheek, thigh, and calf, I knew Mr. Happy was perfectly capable of complete autonomy.

"Are you ready, doctor? We've gotta move." As the latest *Sports Illustrated*

# Big Sucker, Idn'it?

Swimsuit Model of the Year helped me into the MRI scan room, I managed to grab hold of and pseudoapproximate the open rear of the flimsy gown. She positioned me on my back, on the rock-hard, ice-cold table with my knees supported by three pillows.

Any fear of humiliation due to autonomous changes in body parts faded instantly as I caught sight of the tubular tomb into which I would soon be propelled for the MRI. Believe me, the claustrophobic prospect of lying perfectly still, not to mention the throbbing agony down my backside, was enough to eliminate any fleeting concerns I may have had over the potential of exposed portions of my anatomy to Claudia, Vandella, Penelope, Halle, or whomever.

As I began to panic over my upcoming internment, Elle McPherson was putting a tourniquet on my arm. Yeow! That hurts when they twist off your arm hair. I *hate* needles . . . *hate, hate, hate*, needles! She deftly dug in an eighteen-gauge (about the diameter of a sewer pipe), and warned me about a possible "flushed" sensation as the contrast dye ran in. Liquid fire coursed through my veins as she positioned both my arms over my head. The table began to creep toward the black hole of the scanner a few maddening centimeters at a time. I closed my eyes and tried not to picture the inside of this sarcophagus.

It's incredible to me that man has the power to throw a ball accurately, hit one reliably, visually distinguish 3 mm at 20 ft, fly supersonic jet fighters, and play air hockey, but cannot control his own body's manifestations of anxiety. After about two and a half years of lying perfectly still, I began to get restless legs. You know, that sensation you get, usually at night, that you just HAVE TO MOVE! After several stern admonishments from the disembodied voice over the intercom, I was able to force my thoughts away from movement to more pleasant topics, like what a mess my schedule was going to be after returning from surgical leave.

After another fourteen months, the scan was finished. I suffered the further indignity of standing essentially naked before the Athenian goddess and being directed down the hall and to the left to the men's room. I was distinctly conscious of the cool draft on my rear, although I probably only imagined her gaze.

A few minutes later I returned and stepped up into the glassed-off reading room. The computer images were just coming up on the screen, and even a gynecologist could see a large hunk of lumbar disc material protruding into an area for which it was not intended.

"Big sucker, idn't it?" the tech queried before realizing it was I who looked over his shoulder.

"Oh, sorry, Doc," he said taking the ballpoint out of his mouth. "Guess that hurts, huh?"

"Yeah." I grimaced as I shuffled back toward the changing room, right hand still clutching the back of the gown to ensure bottom modesty.

After about eight difficult minutes trying to get dressed while unable to bend over or use my left foot, I emerged once again. The perfectly proportioned and obviously healthy swimsuit model handed me my copy of the films after another wait of fifteen or twenty minutes. She gave me that perky little sand-and-surf smile and said she really hoped I'd be feeling better soon. I felt about eighty-seven years old, and my thoughts of her in a string bikini prancing effortlessly on the beach reinforced my geriatric self-image.

I found my way back to the front desk and finally reestablished contact with the schoolmarm. She directed me to the proper clerk, who finally found my paperwork only to tell me that there was nothing further I needed to do. I waited for a seventy-ish woman—who obviously had more strength than I at the moment—to open the office door, and I hobbled slowly down the corridor to the elevators.

In the neurosurgeon's waiting room, it was deja vu—same grumpy patients, same visual persecution when I was called back to an examining room after only a few moments. While I felt guilty, I was pleased because the pain was getting worse, not better. The nurse took some rudimentary information, laid the proffered films on the desktop, and told me the doctor would be right in.

I remember the room had an exam table that, in my debilitated state, was too high for me to get onto without a step stool. There was none in evidence. There was a small desk and phone but no chair and no windows. I leaned against the exam table and studied the MRI images. It was probably only about twenty minutes later when I started to get annoyed. Couldn't they just pop in and give me a hint as to how long it would be? I decided to kill time by calling my office. If I was going to have disc surgery in the next day or two, it was time to start rescheduling the patients I wouldn't be seeing.

After several minutes on the phone, I made an abortive attempt to get up on the hard leather exam table. The pain was unrelieved in any standing or sitting position, so finally I just lay on the floor. My trusty Seiko now told me we were going on one hour and fifteen minutes. Still no word from Nurse Ratchet. I rolled over, used the table to get to my feet, and opened the door a crack. She was sitting at a desk in a room across the hall eating a jelly donut and drinking coffee. She laughed with someone else in the room who I couldn't see. "Excuse me. Do you have any idea when he'll be here?" My exasperation was unmistakable.

"We'll let you know. Remember, you're an add-in. You know how that is, right?"

I knew how that was, right, but I also know my nurses would be doing something to keep the patient more comfortable—offering a drink, a boost onto the table, or some help to the bathroom.

Dr. Jenkins finally swept into the room just shy of 110 minutes after I had been deposited there. He looked up from his chart, shook my hand, and then helped me onto the exam table. I'm sure he was tied up in surgery, but he didn't mention it.

After I failed each part of the neurological exam, he gave the films a perfunctory review and then offered me two choices: I could live with it and hope it got better or operate on the disc. In light of the fact that I, too, was in a surgical subspecialty, working long hours bent over operating tables, and generally abusing my back, he must have been aware that my current level of functioning would be woefully inadequate. I opted for the surgery.

It was scheduled for three days later. In the interim, no amount of pain reliever, muscle relaxant, or massage seemed of much benefit. When my wife drove me to the hospital at 5:45 a.m. on D-day, it was still pitch black outside. We parked underground, and I hobbled to Admitting.

The first order of business there, and I mean without a "good morning," was to discuss living wills should I end up on life-support indefinitely. Well, my surgery was not a heart-lung transplant, and dying hadn't really crossed my mind. There's got to be a better way to greet the patient than this.

I met with the ubiquitous, too-short, threadbare, open-in-the-back hospital gown again shortly thereafter. My pastor came to visit and pray with me, further reinforcing my perception of approaching doom. As he was preparing to leave, a pretty young nurse (also ubiquitous evidently) came in with an enema bag. After my initial shock and embarrassment, I remembered that after all this was an operation on my back, so I asked to see the doctor's orders. The enema order had not come from my neurosurgeon but from one of my partners. Hardy har har.

Even riding on the gurney while watching the ceiling tiles flash by was an unexpectedly uncomfortable experience. In medical school at Baylor, we had been forced to "experience" being the patient by practicing on each other. We drew each other's blood, inserted nasogastric tubes, placed Foley catheters, did rectal and pelvic exams, etc. But we never thought to whisk each other down a hall flat on our backs on a gurney.

Well, I survived the operation. In fact, I even got to do it again exactly one year later. I was holding two bottles of wine in my right hand—a Christ-

# Big Sucker, Idn'it?

mas gift from a patient—and my briefcase in my left. When it came time to retrieve my car keys, I carefully avoided bending to put down my briefcase. No, instead, I did something much more stupid. I transferred the wine to the crook of my right arm and the briefcase to my right hand, then twisted around and reached into my right pocket with my free left hand. Brilliant! If someone else had been in the parking lot, they could have heard the disc rupture. I screamed, fell to the floor, and got to do it all over again.

"Yuck," is the best way to express my experience as a patient. I don't think it was the pain or the fear or the embarrassment that made it awful. I think it was the helplessness. The patient is truly at the mercy of those who care for him or her. You become an object to which things are done. I believe it's around age two that we seek to become masters of our own environment. Loss of our autonomy at any age beyond that is, at the least, unpleasant, and at the worst, terrifying.

There is no question in my mind that being the patient at some time or another is almost a necessity for developing into an empathetic physician. In my personal case, however, I will strive to keep those instances to a bare minimum.

# Not a Nice Word

---

*Like the perennial lack of sleep, being on call shapes the life of the primary-care physician or surgeon. Every moment of our lives can be and is disrupted by that electronic umbilical cord, the beeper. (For our practice, the beeper became that satanic instrument, the cell phone in 2002.) While this is obviously detrimental to family life, the* call phenomenon *also focuses a doctor's entire life on medicine. Whether good or bad on balance, life on call is an inescapable fact for those who deal with problems that never seem to arise on schedule.*

---

Certainly everyone has been required to stand by for some reason or other during their lives. Perhaps you have awaited the results of a job interview or served as a member of a volunteer fire department or the power company's emergency preparedness team awaiting some catastrophe that wipes out a region's electricity. Maybe you've watched the clock while wondering whether your love-struck teenager would make it home from a date by midnight.

The doctor on call has his own kind of waiting, which produces a strange *je ne sais quoi*. Call it tension, but it's more than that. Being on call does not guarantee that you *will* be called away in the middle of your daughter's first dance recital or your son's first soccer game or out of the choir loft on Sunday morning or even away from your fourteenth wedding anniversary dinner. It means, more fundamentally, the *potential* for those things to happen. Even if they don't, they *might*, and that's the problem. What did Roosevelt say? "We have nothing to fear but fear itself." And the beeper.

"On call" means trapped, cornered, nowhere to run, and nowhere to hide! It's not the unmistakable fact that you might be called into the hospital for an emergency. That alone could be easily dealt with emotionally. It's not even the certainty that you are responsible for the very lives of not only your own patients but your partners' patients as well. That responsibility comes with the territory.

No, it's none of these things. It's somehow the fact that the beeper can go off at the very next instant. That's the killer. It can scare the hell out of you at any time! You can be in stage-four sleep—then suddenly yanked into consciousness with no warning whatsoever. You can have your beeper set on vibrate so that you don't disturb others in the symphony or church or at a lecture. Then—bzzzzzzzz! You look like an idiot when you give an audible start, jump out of your seat for no apparent reason, and apologize to everyone as they readjust to allow you to squeeze by knees, step on toes, and maintain your balance with a quick hand to the shoulder or head of the unsuspecting person sitting one row to the front.

There are other well-known (to doctors) phenomena associated with taking call. For instance, if you are just completing an emergency laparoscopic salpingostomy for an ectopic pregnancy at 4:00 a.m. after sixty-eight hours of a seventy-two-hour weekend call, your beeper will begin its annoying, plaintive cry as you are removing your scrub gown. You were just wondering if you'd get to go home for three to four hours before the new day starts. The page will concern a hysterical young woman in horrible pain and bleeding heavily on her way to the ER. She will be named Hysung Ping and will not speak a word of English. In short, you needn't have worried about going home.

However, frenetic activity is not the callee's worst fate. Almost every physician I know would rather stay continuously busy while on call than simply sit waiting for the other shoe to drop. Physicians go through residencies where they may spend literally years on call every other night. That means you work for about thirty-six hours straight, take maybe twelve off if you're lucky, and then do your thirty-six hours again. You mathematical wizards out there might have figured that comes to roughly 132 hours a week. I bet you didn't realize there were that many hours in the week. Kinda makes forty hours look a bit anemic, doesn't it?

But we can all tell you that as long as you're working every minute, you can get away with it. Sure, you might fall asleep at every red light on the way home, but the old adrenaline's pumpin' if you're taking a bullet out of somebody's pregnant uterus.

No, the problem in residency came when you had thirty minutes of down time at 4:00 a.m. You would fall asleep on the elevator, somnambulate to the call room, and collapse in a heap on the bunk. Revving the engines again when that hideous beeper went off required herculean strength, self-discipline, and dedication.

In private practice, you may not be comatose despite seventy hours on call, because you may have slept for several hours at a stretch throughout the weekend. But you dare not try to go home or to your kid's soccer game or to the circus that night or to that movie you really wanted to see (the last one having been *Lawrence of Arabia*) because of the dreaded hip attachment. If you're swamped, you never have a chance to give it a thought. If you're not terribly busy, it's torture.

I should also mention some other well-known call phenomena. I don't care what the American College of Obstetrics and Gynecology study showed; all of us OBs know that the moon's gravitational force ruptures membranes. Why is this so hard to believe? After all, the moon tosses around multiple quadrillion tons of ocean water without perceptible effort twice each day. Surely a few liters of amniotic fluid should pose little challenge for the lunar forces.

# Not a Nice Word

And what about the *hex*? You have not left the hospital building for fifty-six hours. You have just completed a particularly nerve-wracking, mid-forceps delivery, and it was absolutely the last thing you had to do, and someone asks you if you have anyone else on the way in. Well, forget it; you are hosed. Sometimes, if you pretend not to have heard the question and you're convincing, the obstetric gods will consider a reprieve. This, however, is extremely rare. Usually, your beeper senses the question and initiates its incessant buzzing or beeping instantaneously. Occasionally, even your spouse, in his/her ardent desire to have you come home, will err and innocently ask the fatal question. C'est la vie!

It doesn't matter if you have a conference to attend in the Virgin Islands or you're on the vacation you've waited eight years to enjoy and planned six months in advance. Some emergency with someone, somewhere, will alter the schedule such that you draw the black bean. You just have to take call right then.

Now, you say, that has to work both ways. There must be times that a doctor needs to get off, and others alter their schedule to make it possible. Well, that must be the case, but I'll be damned if any of us can ever remember the last time that happened.

I can hear the objections. "Oh, quit griping! You picked this for a living, didn't you?"

Well, not exactly. When you apply to medical school, the counselors skip over the part about no sleep, the ugly specter of too many attorneys without enough to eat, the physical attachment to the obnoxious little box on your hip, the unimaginably political bureaucracies called hospitals, and the fact that your children ask for identification before they'll open the front door for you.

But they say that taking call builds character. I suppose in a way it does. It certainly drives home the meaning of the word *responsibility* in one context. Some of us, however, took marriage vows that antedated our taking the Hippocratic oath. While responsibility may well be learned along the path to becoming a reputable physician, it must also be applied to the role of husband and father. The balance is often extremely precarious. The high divorce rate among physicians is often quoted as evidence for their misplaced loyalties but usually not as evidence for the total lack thereof. Their loyalties just end up right where they were placed on the first day of medical school with the patient first, last, and foremost.

I firmly believe that the most effective physician is one who has a secure and rewarding family life. His family benefits from his presence almost as much as he benefits from their support. Fostering this environment takes time and learning. It took me more than six years as a physician to finally understand that when my home number came up on the digital beeper or cell phone, I needed to make the call the top priority rather than the bottom.

So "call" is truly a four-letter word. We learn to deal with it as a fact of life, but we never really like it. All of us know deep inside our beings that pagers and cell phones are instruments of the devil. But, in spite of call, and perhaps partially because of call, we learn that responsibility lies at the heart of a successful life.

# The Bad Disease

*We've alluded before to the fallible nature of physicians. We need to realize that errors with sweeping consequences can come in many forms. But a strong physician-patient relationship can ameliorate the effects of such errors. In fact, as will be mentioned in "Danger," it is the strength of such a relationship that can avert many of these errors, and the lack of such a relationship that might allow things to fall through the cracks.*

It was an even busier morning than usual. The bright April sunshine streamed in through the exam room windows. Moving splotches of gold danced over the counters, cabinets, and exam tables. Outside it was cool and breezy, a gorgeous day. All of my patients probably wished they were someplace else, but it was unusual for me to wish that I was too.

As I exited the exam room and prepared to dictate my visit notes, I was thinking about the fact that my weekend off and this phenomenal weather might actually coincide, defying known physical laws of obstetrics. Then I caught a glimpse of my nurse putting one of those sticky notes where I couldn't possibly miss it. That almost always meant trouble. My good mood vaporized.

The note simply said, "Call Sarah, urgent" with a phone number. Usually that kind of note would be annoying: which Sarah? What was the problem? Where was her chart? But it wasn't annoyance I felt this time. And I knew perfectly well which Sarah. What could possibly be urgent to a person in her almost unimaginable position?

Sarah was a thirty-eight-year-old clinical psychologist married to a corporate attorney. Married for over fifteen years, they were happy but infertile. Over the course of the last several years they had endured the entire gamut of infertility tests and procedures. Now they had become the living embodiment of the term "advanced reproductive technology," and they were ecstatic after the discovery of their twin pregnancy.

While Sarah was technically of advanced maternal age, and thus at some increased risk for various complications, in general she was the optimum candidate for pregnancy at this time of life. Strong, healthy, and trim, Sarah balanced her busy work schedule by swimming up to 3,000 meters a day, a near perfect exercise for pregnancy, even for women with multiple gestations.

Educated about her primary risks of preterm labor and preeclampsia or toxemia, Sarah was totally in tune with her body. She recognized her own uterine contractions, even the subtle ones barely detected on the monitor. She combined her exercise with an optimum diet, and her blood pressure had remained low-normal throughout the pregnancy. Her pelvic ultrasound at eighteen weeks had shown two girls, both growing at the same rate and without abnormality. In short, she had done "swimmingly" through her first twenty-six weeks of gestation.

She had called around midnight at the start of her twenty-seventh week, complaining of excruciating left flank pain. When I met her about 1:00 a.m. at labor and delivery, I knew there was something serious going on. Her husband was standing on the far side of the bed holding Sarah in his arms. She was twisted toward him and half sitting, the lower half of her body on the bed.

She was still for just that one moment when I walked in, her teeth clenched, her face a mask of agony, her arms wrapped around her husband's neck. Immediately thereafter she resumed her writhing, pushing away from her husband and falling full onto the bed. She rolled back and forth, pleading and screaming for relief through tears of pain.

Anyone who has ever passed a kidney stone, or taken care of anyone who did, recognizes the typical presentation. Almost any other kind of intra-abdominal emergency, from a ruptured appendix to a ruptured cyst or ectopic pregnancy, will cause the patient to curl up on her side and lie as still as possible. With a kidney stone, the patient usually does a good imitation of a large-mouth bass flopping around on the dock. (One diagnostic test for abdominal pain is to "accidentally" jostle the gurney on which the patient is lying and observe the reaction. The kidney stone patient won't notice, but the intra-abdominal catastrophe patient will scream bloody murder.)

But I knew Sarah. I knew her tears were not all pain but frustration as well. If there was one thing she didn't like, it was losing control. As a clinical psychologist, she dealt with patients whose problems ran the gamut from the mundane young-mother neuroses to the dangerous borderline personalities. Most of the time, Sarah couldn't afford to do anything other than run steady and true on an even keel. To be this out of control was painful physically and emotionally.

After some reassurance about the safety of narcotic pain relievers at twenty-seven weeks of pregnancy and the importance of avoiding a seriously preterm twin delivery at almost any cost, Sarah agreed to IV morphine. Her pelvic exam was not too worrisome with respect to cervical change, and despite her agonized thrashing about, delivery did not look to be an immediate concern. We made plans for the usual kidney ultrasound and one shot of IVP (intravenous pyelogram), which I felt would surely reveal her kidney stone.

Her pain improved markedly after the morphine. Her urine showed no blood whatsoever. By two hours after arrival, she had no pain at all. While this was somewhat atypical of a stone, we agreed to not pursue any further testing unless there was a recurrent episode. We gave her the usual instruction about how to strain her urine, since she had probably passed the stone into her bladder when the pain stopped, and sent her home with some prophylactic antibiotics.

I saw Sarah the following week, and except for a dull, intermittent ache in the flank, she was doing fine. The twins continued to grow concordantly (at the same rate), and we discussed her cutting back a bit at the office. We also took the necessary steps to set up twice-per-day home uterine contraction monitoring via a corporation to which Sarah could transfer her monitoring strips over the phone. The subsequent record could be faxed to us as needed, or more usually, a computer graphic was produced weekly to indicate any patterns of increasingly frequent contractions.

It was only three days later when I saw her again. Unfortunately, to my consternation, it was in a fourth-floor room on the high-risk OB wing. Her hair was disheveled and soaked from perspiration. She was paler than usual, if that's possible for a redhead. The effect of the narcotics had given her hazel eyes a glazed appearance in the dimly lit room. Her small swimmer's frame, despite the broad shoulders, looked overwhelmed by the size of her protuberant belly. Her husband, Harold, was sitting on the other side of the bed holding her left hand in both of his. He was balding and of medium build, had glasses, and looked worried. Maybe a little angry, but not overtly so.

My associate had admitted her this time. She'd come in around 3:00 a.m. (of course) with the same violently intense flank pain. Sarah had continued to swim long distances each day, and I had agreed. But the pain seemed totally unrelated to physical activity. It had awakened her from a sound sleep and had come on like a freight train, easing for a while but then returning in relentless waves. My partner had already set her up for the ultrasound and the X-ray, and they were coming to get her soon.

By the time I saw her, the pain was once again on the way to resolution, much as it had been ten days previously. But as agreed, I felt it important to get to the bottom of this now. Again her urine was negative for blood or infection. Her white blood count was normal. She had no fever. Her symptoms could go along with pyelonephritis or kidney infection; however, her lab work was incompatible. A kidney stone still seemed the most likely etiology of her pain.

While we talked and Harold took what was to become a long list of notes on a legal pad, the X-ray tech arrived with the gurney to take her down into the bowels of the hospital, through the tunnel across the parking lot, and then up into the main building where most of the imaging equipment was located. I rode the elevator down with them and gave her a quick hug when we reached my floor, promising to come discuss the results with her as soon as I had them.

It was several hours later when I walked into their room. She was in bed but fully dressed, holding a four-by-four inch gauze over the site where her IV had just been removed. Pain obviously gone, she gave her trademark big smile.

"So, am I outta here? Did they see the stone?"

Her face changed slowly as she looked at mine. Harold took his feet down off the bed and muted the TV with the remote. Without comment, he picked up his legal pad off the window ledge.

"It doesn't look like a stone, Sarah. There appears to be a growth on your left kidney of some sort. This one looks like it might be fairly large, since it distorts the image of the ureter, but we'll need a CAT scan or MRI to get a better look." Now Sarah and Harold are well-read, intelligent people, and the term *growth* was pretty transparent to them.

"Are you telling me that I have a kidney tumor?"

"You certainly might, or at least the two studies you had today were suggestive of that. But even if it's true, malignant tumors of the kidney in your age group are almost unheard of. Our problem is going to be keeping your babies on the inside until they're ready to breathe on their own."

Sarah was reaching for a tissue, the first shiny tears trickling from the corners of her eyes. Harold spoke for the first time.

"How do you know for a fact that it's not malignant?" he said, pen poised over his legal pad.

"First, we need a urology consult, and I imagine he'll want a tissue diagnosis. By that I would normally mean a needle biopsy, but we really should talk to urology first and follow up on the results of the CAT scan I have scheduled tomorrow."

"But isn't a biopsy dangerous? I mean, what about bleeding? What about the twins? Could there be something wrong with them too? Could this deal be hereditary? What if it is *cancer*? If it is, I want it *out* right now! No waiting for . . ." He was getting more and more excited as each new possibility occurred to him.

"Hold on there a minute!" I interrupted. "We don't know she has a tumor. If she does, it is in all probability benign and won't affect anything except possibly to further increase her risk of preterm labor. If that is the case, and she goes into preterm labor, we have medicines to deal with that."

I sat on the end of her bed and grabbed a tennis-shoed foot.

"I want you to stay off of these for awhile. We can do the CAT scan as an outpatient, and then you can see my buddy the urologist the following day. It was about time for you to quit work in any event." I gave her foot a good-natured dog shake. "Look, it's gonna be alright. If something bad happened it could hurt my reputation, and I'll not have that!" It got a little smile out of her. Her husband did not look terribly reassured.

I don't believe she even got the CAT scan as an outpatient. The pain returned the next night, and she was right back on the high-risk antepartum unit. I do remember that the CAT scan did not look like the usual fatty benign renal tumor. In fact, the radiologist told me that it looked quite a bit like the "bad disease." The urologist and I agreed that an MRI would be even more helpful.

The evening after the MRI, I spent nearly an hour in Sarah's room. Harold was much calmer than initially, and his questions were logical and well thought out. Sarah was unusually quiet, and although her questions were less frequent, they always centered around the twins. It rapidly became clear that slightly different priorities were emerging.

Harold cut to the chase.

"So, there definitely is a large tumor in the left kidney, and it doesn't look like the kind of benign tumor that would be more common in her age group?"

"That is true," I said simply.

"Okay, let's take the worst-case scenario. Let's just assume this is cancer. What do we do?" Sarah was crying quietly again. The lights in the room were off and the sky was in that final gray stage before true darkness, a good hour after sunset. The parking lot lights were stark; they silhouetted Harold in his position on the windowsill, his legal pad over one crossed leg.

"We'll have to talk more with Brian (the urologist), but I do know this kidney will have to be removed. It is extremely unlikely that this tumor could be removed and also save any normal kidney. First, there is now little function in the involved kidney, and the surgery to remove the entire kidney would be safer, quicker, and with less blood loss than trying just to remove the tumor. Whether or not the tumor is . . . "

"When?" Sarah said. "Just, when?"

There was one of those awkward silences. All I could tell them for sure was that surgery stood an extremely high chance of precipitating preterm labor. Twins at twenty-eight weeks do better now than ever before in NICUs (neonatal intensive care units), but they also die 10–20% of the time and are permanently damaged in some way a greater percentage of time than that. I recommended that we wait at least another month until thirty-two weeks if possible. That would give the twins an excellent chance of undamaged survival, even if Sarah went into preterm labor.

"Why not wait until the twins are really ready and do both surgeries at the same time? Wouldn't that be best for the twins?" Sarah wanted to know. Almost without hesitation, Harold asked if it wouldn't be better for Sarah to get it out as soon as possible. Like tomorrow, for instance.

How's this for a potential no-win situation? Do a nephrectomy (removal of the kidney) ASAP, and possibly lose twins who were ten years in the making. Given the couple's infertility and age, that might close the book on their chance to reproduce. The other choice was to delay the surgery and deal with the risk for preterm labor, which was already worsening, in the hope of getting healthy twins, but possibly leaving the patient's malignancy to spread over the next four to six weeks.

I left the room with a clear message from the patient—do what must be done to give the twins the best chance. I left the room with a clear message from the patient's husband—do what must be done to save my wife's life.

After further discussion with the urologist and his partners, we decided that the odds were still way in favor of this being a benign tumor. Consequently, I would do what was necessary to avoid delivery until thirty-four weeks. We would then perform a cesarean section; the twins would have an excellent chance; We would delay removal of the kidney until six weeks postpartum when her blood volume had recovered.

Harold was difficult to convince. Our argument was that, if malignant, despite the lack of distant metastases, a tumor this size would surely have already ruptured the renal capsule, and delay in removal would do little to prolong the inevitable. Harold wasn't buying it.

As it turned out, after discharge, Harold and Sarah got a second opinion at the medical school. The chief of urology there felt that there was a significant chance of malignancy with this tumor's appearance, and he recommended immediate removal.

We resolved the controversy the only way we could—the way all men do in the long run. We did what we were told—Harold by his wife, me by my patient. We agreed to delay the surgery until at least thirty-two weeks, giving the twins a good chance at normalcy if we were forced to deliver them, but hopefully maintain the pregnancy for at least another month after the nephrectomy.

Sarah continued to swim over the next several weeks despite increasing discomfort. She continued to be the model patient, and her uterine contractions, while increasingly frequent, were not enough to prove dangerous.

OOO

I don't think I'll ever forget the image of a small-framed, naked woman with a huge abdomen lying halfway on her back and halfway on her side, chest arched unnaturally over a roll. Her arms were extended over her head, an endotracheal tube taped into her mouth, her eyes taped closed. Fetal heart tones were fine as we prepped and draped her flank.

The surgery to remove the kidney went well. The pathology did not. There is no easy way to deliver the news that someone has what everyone prayed they did not. There is no easy way to tell a loving, devoted husband that his mate has an incurable cancer. It is a death knell. It is the end of the world as he knows it. It is a betrayal, in a way. It is incomprehensible. We told Harold we would have to await the final pathology, but the frozen section looked very worrisome. We told him that the surgery had gone as well as could be expected. He was tearful and silent.

Sarah went to the antepartum ICU. She was on a special subcutaneous terbutaline pump to keep her contractions under control. There was an epidural in place to help with post-op pain. As it turned out, it was too low to be very helpful, and her next few days were miserable. She was in and out of a narcotic stupor and battling with IVs, bladder catheter, nausea, itching, and almost unimaginable discomfort at thirty-two weeks with twins *and* a foot-long, muscle-splitting flank incision.

# Disrobe Completely

Then came a chain of snafus. Three days after the operation, a well-meaning floor nurse called the psychiatry social worker because Sarah had been difficult and demanding since surgery. The floor nurse neglected to ask either me or the urologist if this was okay; in fact, neither of us had yet been informed of the final path report, which had just come back. The social worker read the report, then interrupted Sarah's visit with a friend, asked the visitor to leave, and questioned Sarah as to how she might help her deal with her anger.

"Anger about what?" Sarah asked.

"Why, your anger about your cancer, of course!"

I got there about ten minutes later, having told my nurse to cancel the remaining two hours of the afternoon. Sarah was inconsolable. In a cowardly sort of fashion, I felt that the situation was now much easier for me. I sat on the bed and held Sarah in my arms as she rocked back and forth like a small child. She reminded me of my own little girl when I would try to quiet the wracking sobs which accompanied a particularly frightening nightmare.

In the ensuing days, I spent many more hours with the two of them. While urology would give them the straight facts, I would come by to reinterpret them in a better light. When they told her it was a particularly rare form of renal sarcoma, I would tell her at least it hadn't broken through the renal capsule. When they told her it could already have spread elsewhere through her bloodstream, I told her there was no evidence that it had, and as far as anyone but God knew, she might well already be cured.

We delayed discussion of further therapy until after her delivery. She did well once off the preterm labor medicines; just as soon as she had almost fully recovered from her flank incision, it was time for her cesarean section. We got all the way to thirty-six weeks, and twin girls were born without a hitch.

How can one describe the melancholy surrounding the joyful delivery of long-awaited twins to a loving mother who has been told there is less than a 5% chance that she will witness their second birthday? In the weeks that followed, Sarah began a journal and videotapes of instructions for the girls to be played as they reached anticipated birthdays and expected goals all the way to adulthood. She tried to think of herself as cured and take one day at a time, but it was difficult in light of the facts she faced. The local chemotherapy doctors told her there was no effective regimen for her disease and recommended no treatment unless metastases showed up. Sarah and Harold both wanted the most aggressive treatment available. I agreed they should go to M.D. Anderson in Houston for a second opinion.

○○○

When I saw the sticky note, I just couldn't imagine what was urgent. Surely she had not already developed a distant symptom, and it was too far out from her C-section to be a surgical complication. We had spoken only two days ago on her return from Houston. The doctors there agreed that the only treatment would be toxic, experimental, unlikely to have any benefit, and would adversely affect large blocks of her few remaining healthy months. What could possibly be urgent?

I dialed the phone and braced myself.

"Hi, gorgeous! What's so urgent?" I tried to be my usual jovial self.

"I'm not gonna die. How's that for urgent!" You could just see her beaming.

"Excuse me?" I couldn't hide my bewilderment.

"You were right to begin with. You told me it wasn't gonna be cancer before the surgery. Then you told me to think cured afterwards." She was giddy.

"I'm still lost, Sarah."

"M.D. Anderson just called. They reviewed the slides. I don't have cancer. They've all reviewed them down there and nobody thinks it's malignant!"

"That's fantastic!" I screamed, drawing inquiring looks from my patient checking out, the receptionist, and the nurse. "I guess this means a little boo-boo in our path department though, huh?"

"Yeah. But it's hard to be angry right now. Apparently it's a rare type of tumor that looked confusing under the microscope. But 'Oops' is a lot easier when it's 'Oops, no cancer!' So can you believe it?"

"I believe it, Sarah. Go swim some laps. I've got new energy for work!"

The sun was still streaming in the windows. It really was springtime after all. Once more I had learned that *nothing* is written in stone; it's okay to count my chicks before they hatch; it's not over 'til the fat lady sings; the rain in Spain falls mainly on the plain; whiskers on kittens and blue satin sashes are among my favorite things—and it really does help to whistle a happy tune whenever you feel afraid.

○○○

The microscope slides, as it turns out, were not confusing in the least; they were the wrong slides. Apparently the pathologist had mixed in some slides on a rare type of renal sarcoma for an upcoming lecture with the patient's actual slides by mistake. Did Sarah succomb to the urgings of everyone she ran into and sue everyone involved? Nope. She had a party, the theme of which was "celebrating life." She invited everyone involved in her care, including the pathologist.

# A Little Bit in Love

*Being a physician is not just another job. It's a commitment to doing the utmost to maintain and restore the health of our patients—the health that is not merely physical or emotional but the interweaving of both that makes people what they are when they're at their best.*

*The following is a very personal experience. I feel I can relate it now in part because it happened so long ago, and also because I feel so strongly that the essence of the physician-patient relationship is in grave danger in this country today. I don't expect that the depth of feeling I recall here could—or should—be brought to a doctor's every relationship with a patient. But I do know that in this patient's ordeal, I learned about loss. I learned about compassion. I learned about love in a real sense. And I learned that averting suffering is a worthy goal in life.*

She was twenty-six, maybe twenty-seven years old. She didn't look it, of course, lying there soaked in sweat. Her hospital gown clung to her rail-thin frame as though only fossilized remains were concealed. Her once-porcelain skin was bruised horribly; every inch of her neck and forearms was covered with splotches of purple, green, and yellow. Her most recent IV site was, I think she knew, to be her final one. The bulky bandage on her left upper chest protruded awkwardly from the neck of the faded blue gown. The subclavian IV tubing lay as limp as her spirit across the pillow. No, she didn't look twenty-six. But it wasn't that she looked older, either. She just didn't look right. She just didn't look right at all.

Her long brown hair had long since been lost. Only those of us who had seen her in years past could even visualize the beautiful girl she had been. The chemotherapy had seemed to go on forever. Methotrexate, cytoxan, adriamy-cin (the Red Death, we called it): she'd had it all in multiple courses. This last time in, though, was the worst. Maybe it was the worst because of the bleed into her head with the resulting loss of movement on the left side, or maybe because of the radiation to her already denuded scalp, but surely because she and all the rest of us knew she wouldn't be leaving the hospital again.

It had happened like most cases of fatal choriocarcinoma. A happy, bright, optimistic woman of twenty-three had become pregnant a little before she had planned. She and her boyfriend had decided to keep the baby and commit their lives to each other, but as fate would have it, the young lady began spotting and cramping at about seven weeks gestation and subsequently lost the pregnancy.

Because she was so early on when the spotting began, the doctor had told her bed rest was her only option. Despite compliance, her cramping and bleeding rapidly worsened one night. The girl was frightened and just ready to head for the emergency room when the cramping stopped abruptly and the bleeding tailed off to only spotting again. She called the doctor, who told her that she had probably passed all the tissue and completed her miscarriage. Had she saved the tissue? Well, no. No one had told her that was important. He reassured her that it was okay, but he needed to see her back in the office in three to four weeks for a follow-up.

Her boyfriend could hardly hide his relief at the turn of events. She, on the other hand, was devastated. How could the loss of the life they had made together mean so little to him? He said that wasn't it. She wasn't being fair, and he was just being realistic. She told him to get the hell out. He did.

# A Little Bit in Love

The loss of her pregnancy as well as her dream of the handsome prince was almost too much to bear. Her depression lasted for several months, but with the love and support of her parents and her friends, she began to recover in the next six months. Her parents owned a successful winery in Sonoma and, consequently, were quite well off. They sent her and her girlfriend on a six-week tour of Europe, where they used their Eurail passes to extinction. They did Portugal, Spain, France, and Italy, then left the coast to take in Switzerland, Austria, Germany, Holland, and Denmark, and then back to London. Her only regret was not getting to see the Greek isles. But there was always time for that, right?

The appointment. That follow-up appointment—she'd forgotten all about that. Now it had been over a year. She really should go back to see him, and her periods hadn't really been all that regular, had they? In fact, she couldn't really remember when the last one had occurred. Wasn't it back in the summer, before she'd left for Europe? Oh well, she'd just make an appointment now and get in to see him.

The doctor had been pleasant enough. Hadn't she gotten the letters he'd sent her about follow-up? No? Well, we'll just set things right today. Did she have a current sexual partner? No? No one since before the miscarriage? She didn't really know when her last period was?

His exam had been routine. He told her that he felt nothing abnormal. But would she mind leaving a urine specimen in the bathroom off the exam room?

She was writing her check at the front desk when the doctor came up beside her and gently placed his left hand on her forearm. Could she step into the office just for a second? He had something they needed to discuss.

She told me that she often thought of that afternoon. She had sat across the desk from him. The guest chair had faced west, but she could gaze out the picture windows to the north and catch a magnificent view of the bay. The sunlight was streaming over the white caps, bouncing off the straight white walls of Alcatraz, and bathing the vast expanse of green between the marina and the yacht club in a golden afternoon glow. The whole window framed an idyllic scene, which she remembered as a rainbow palette of color given life by the wind, with soaring gulls, billowing sails, and ocean spray on the breakwaters.

He was telling her that her pregnancy test was positive. She told me that she clearly remembered giggling inside, anticipating his retraction when he learned of her celibacy since the miscarriage. Then, as she glanced out the window again, she remembered that he already had asked about that. She started to get a little scared with the realization that the test wasn't in error.

After the word *cancer*, she pretty much tuned out everything. She hadn't meant to, but she'd suddenly remembered the Greek isles and the look on her boyfriend's face the first time they had made love and the fact that she hadn't sent either of her parents cards for Mother's Day or Father's Day this year. These things she told to me.

Eventually she was to fully understand what gestational trophoblastic disease entailed. There were no blood pregnancy assays for human chorionic gonadotropin (hCG—the pregnancy hormone) back then. The urine tests were also markedly less sensitive. Today, a positive pregnancy test will pick up only 25 mIU of hCG in the urine, and this only ten days after conception. Back then, the urine tests were sensitive to about 10,000 mIU of hCG, or four-hundred-fold less sensitive. They would pick up a normal pregnancy no earlier than six weeks from the last period or about thirty days after conception. Unfortunately for the patient, this meant that the presence of a gestational trophoblastic neoplasm (GTN) could not be detected until it was advanced enough to produce relatively high levels of hCG, its marker hormone.

You see, GTN is a particularly tragic trick of fate. It only develops after a spontaneous miscarriage, a genetically abnormal pregnancy called a mole, or rarely after term pregnancy. The placenta is normally an invasive organ. No one yet understands why it normally halts its invasion of the human female when partially burrowed in the wall of the uterus.

As one in fifty Asian women and one in one thousand Caucasian woman know, however, it doesn't always stop.

The chorion, or outer layer of the placental tissue, may become abnormally aggressive, grow through the wall of the uterus, and/or spread its malignant cells to distant parts of the body, such as the lung, liver and brain. Prior to the 1960s, this disease was uniformly and rapidly fatal. By 1975, it was almost completely curable with drugs if detected early. But only *if* detected early.

Today, patients with this disease might be handled largely as outpatients, but at that time, it was routine to admit them for a full work-up. She arrived in old bell-bottom jeans and a peasant blouse, carrying a floral carpet bag containing the worldly possessions she thought essential for such a venture. I had seen her walk by the nurses' station from the elevator, accompanied by a statuesque, middle-aged woman in a stunning red dress who wore jewelry in a way that said she was quite accustomed to such luxuries.

It was that first day that I was assigned to her care as a second-year resident. We were at the university hospital up on the hill overlooking Kezar Stadium and Golden Gate Park beyond. She'd had her blood drawn already and had just returned from X-ray when I stepped in. She was an impossibly beautiful girl, or maybe I've just made her that way in my memory. She sat on the edge of the bed, clutching a large, once white, shabby teddy bear to her chest.

She looked up as I entered the room, flipping her long chestnut hair over her shoulder with just a toss of her head. (They must teach beautiful girls how to do that just right somewhere; oh yeah, in kindergarten.) Her hazel eyes seemed to sparkle, perhaps a little moist, as they caught the late afternoon sun through the window. She was now attired in the infamous, faded, blue hospital gown, open to the rear, but had managed to hang on to her tight bell-bottoms.

# Disrobe Completely

I introduced myself to her and her mother and asked if this was a good time to talk to her for a few minutes. Her mother commented that I looked awfully young. The patient, almost whispering, said that any time was a good time now, wasn't it? The mother reached out and put her hand on her daughter's arm. "Stop that, honey. It's gonna work out, you'll see." Her glance said she wasn't that sure of her words or of me.

The rest of that interview was pretty much like any other where a parent is present, i.e., the mother constantly answered questions directed at her daughter, continuing her lifelong role as protector. It was impossible to inject any levity into the situation. But despite the patient's intermittent crying, she and I shared a private smile at the expense of her mother when the lady turned her attention to rooting through her oversized purse for some vaccination records.

As any doctor might have expected, the chest X-ray showed multiple cannon ball metastases throughout the lung fields. Her urine collection showed levels well over the 100,000 mark required to assign her to the poor prognosis group. By the time the next day's CAT scan results were available, it was no surprise to anyone that her liver was a minefield as well. Only the brain scan was normal.

Despite this troubling picture, we were able to give the patient some hope. People with this disease do respond remarkably well to modern chemotherapy. Because no gross tumor could be imaged in the uterus and a D&C was unrevealing, surgery was not proposed as part of her treatment. In fact, the appearance of her metastases were so classic that biopsy data was not even deemed necessary before starting treatment.

○○○

I was on the oncology service for three months, so I managed to see her over several hospitalizations. She'd be in for four to six days, home for a week or two, and back again for treatment.

We residents mixed the Red Death ourselves so as to absolve the nurses of any responsibility should there be a dosing error. We mixed it under a vacuum vented hood with masks and gloves on, so that not even the fumes of the potent agent could reach our tissues. It always struck me as bizarre to take all these precautions against any possible accidental exposure, and then march into this young woman's room, hook up her IV, and pump this toxin directly into her veins with a smile on my face.

She took it quite well. After her initial terror, she would joke with me about how little she feared chemo, having been forced to drink the family's wine for nearly three decades! But the vomiting was God-awful, and the phenothiazine derivatives (antinausea medications) never really helped unless we gave her enough to knock her out for a few hours. Often, I would be rushing to finish one of the hundreds of tasks required daily to evaluate and treat the thirty to forty cancer patients on the floor at any one time when I would peek in her door and find her sleeping on her side with her arms around that ragged bear. I remember feeling guilty that I found myself praying for her recovery and not for any of the other patients in my charge, most of whom were thirty to fifty years her senior.

It only took one admission for me to realize I was looking forward to her next. She responded better than we could have hoped, her hCG dropping quickly and dramatically after the first few treatments. Her chest X-ray cleared, her liver enzymes returned to normal, and those of us new and naive enough began to feel proud of ourselves for defeating this scourge.

She looked just as gorgeous without any hair to me. She used to love to return to the floor unscheduled, wearing a new wig and sunglasses, and fool the nurses who knew her so well into believing she was whoever she claimed to be that day.

I never saw her tearful again after that first day. Never. Even after the third and fourth relapses over two years later, she maintained her ebullient determination. Always her hCG titers would drop, but never back to the normal range, and each time the descent was slower. We used to present her graphs in conference as examples of the relentless nature of the disease.

While the chemotherapy only took a few days, her weakened immune system always permitted some viral or bacterial invader to take up residence briefly before being evicted by antibiotics. Thus her hospital stays toward the spring of 1984 became longer; the next to last time she came, she was hospitalized for two weeks.

Her friends stopped visiting toward the end. I don't know whether their lives had forced them to move on, or they just couldn't stand to watch death's inexorable approach. Incredibly, I found myself frequently stopping to sit with her at the end of a gruesome day to cheer *myself* up. Sometimes we'd sit for forty-five minutes and talk of our respective plans. She'd always ask after my wife. When I'd drag myself into her room after seventy-two hours awake, she'd reassure me that one day it would all be worth it. She'd talk of her plans for the Greek isles, finally deciding that living there would be better than just visiting. So she worked out an elaborate schedule for the next summer that would end with her finding some Greek god and trampling grapes naked on a hillside in the sun.

When I left her room that Friday after the stroke, I couldn't stop crying. I'd controlled myself in the room and even laughed when she summoned her miniscule strength to imitate the creature from the black lagoon, drawing attention to the drooping left side of her once pretty face. We'd held hands most of that last visit. Her family was nowhere to be seen, but it's possible that I had simply missed their visits.

I told her I still wanted to see her winery before she headed for Greece next summer. She promised me a tour and attempted a smile. I don't know if either of us really knew we'd never see the other again, but I kissed her forehead as I snuggled her bear up against her. She closed her eyes and said she needed a nap.

I was off that weekend. I remember we went up to Stinson Beach and basked in the sun and the sea air. In retrospect, I'm not sure I even thought of her much that Saturday at the beach. I was too busy soaking up life for myself.

Monday, she was gone. I went by her room in the morning around 7:00 a.m. expecting to see that old bear and his lifelong charge, and, instead, found an emaciated elderly Chinese woman with terminal ovarian cancer. At first I thought perhaps she'd been moved to the ICU for life support. But then I realized she would never have permitted that.

When I got home that night about 9:00 p.m., there was a case of wine on the coffee table. My wife wondered who it was from. The tag said simply that this was "just in case we didn't get a chance to take that tour." I sank to the couch and, in a quite unmanly fashion, burst into tears. My wife pulled my head to her lap as I fell over and surrendered to the sobs.

I guess, maybe, I was a little bit in love with her.

Her name was Samantha.

# Sacred Trust

*While physicians deal with both the technical and the emotional aspects of their patients' care, they must also deal with constraints placed on them by the very structure of that physician-patient relationship. Preserving confidentiality is of course paramount to a trusting relationship, but much as it can with attorney-client privilege, that confidentiality can lead one into ethical dilemmas.*

*Many of these dilemmas might seem more easily resolved by breaching the confidence in order to prevent further injury, but the doctor must choose, almost without fail, to err in favor of the sacred trust he has established with his charge via the Hippocratic oath.*

My mistake was in agreeing to see the patient in the first place. Seeing your wife's best friend professionally is almost, but not quite, as stupid as seeing your wife professionally. While it may be unwise *a priori*, it is particularly unwise in a situation such as this one.

After all, my first helpful little bit of medical advice for Sharon had come several years ago when her little boy, then four, had flown off of his new swing set like an unguided missile. My wife and I had the misfortune of being there in the backyard at the time.

Being the swell guy that I am, I cursorily examined the screaming child and assured his mother that neither of her son's injured arms was fractured. Apparently my gynecologic training had obliterated any memories of the greenstick fractures common in toddlers who fall onto their outstretched arms. Needless to say, after a sleepless night of whimpering, a set of X-rays, and an exam by a qualified pediatric orthopedic surgeon, Kevin got to wear casts on both arms for the next six weeks.

While our relationship remained cordial, the red flags should have gone up when my wife discovered that her friend's recent insurance switch did not allow her to see the Ob/Gyn she had seen for years and suggested that she see me instead. Kevin was five by then, and our friends were anxious to multiply but had evidently been having difficulty with the "be fruitful" part. Well, again like the swell guy that I am, I offered to see Sharon for insurance only, fully realizing that this probably meant free where infertility was concerned.

In the course of the first visit, Sharon's history revealed Kevin to be a miracle baby in that her husband's semen analysis proved him to be sterile. There must have been some reason for the evaporation of his sperm-making capabilities, but none was offered.

Right there, had this not been my wife's best friend, I would have questioned her story. But no, I blindly accepted this history as the Gospel. A discussion of donor insemination ensued, and shortly thereafter, arrangements were made for frozen donor insemination from a reputable national bank. The sperm from the donor whose description Sharon and her husband had chosen was flown into town in liquid nitrogen, thawed, and placed high in the uterus via a transcervical catheter on the appropriate day before and again on the day after ovulation. This was done since the sperm can live in the female genital tract for forty-eight to seventy-two hours while the egg only survives for up to twenty-four hours. After I confirmed the egg's readiness with vaginal ultrasound, ovulation was induced by injection of the hormone that signals egg release.

Again, the first cycle should have been a warning of bad karma. Naturally, the appropriate day had fallen on a weekend, so that I had given the shot personally rather than the nurse. Sharon's injection site became extremely red and swollen like none other I had ever seen. Well, it was either an allergic reaction to the serum or an abscess. I treated her with oral antibiotics, and it resolved over several painful days, while I reassured Sharon as to the infinitesimal possibility of it happening again.

Of course, it did happen again the following cycle, and luckily my embarrassment was lessened by the fact that during this cycle she conceived. Everyone was ecstatic! Errors of judgment with respect to greenstick fractures were forgotten by all. Now, like the swell guy I am, I agreed to continue seeing Sharon as an obstetric patient. Her husband had just lost his job. Insurance-only status saved them money, and so, of course, I agreed to see her, despite feeling vaguely uncomfortable.

Her first OB visit was like thousands of others. Ultrasound revealed a 16 mm fetus with a beating heart, and we were all thrilled. We went through the usual first OB visit discussions covering review of medications, diet, exercise, travel, sex, and antenatal testing when appropriate. She had the usual pap smear, group B-strep culture, and routine labs. All went well. Everybody was happy and relieved.

Then her HIV test came back positive. Whoa, what did you just say? Your wife's best friend's HIV test came back positive? Your wife's monogamous, God-fearing, never-had-a-blood-transfusion, pure-as-the-driven-snow best friend's HIV test came back positive?

Read major problem here. Read patient confidentiality above all else. Read a terrified young woman who can't explain to her best friend why she seems to be crying all the time. Read a doctor who can't tell his wife why her best friend seems to be crying all the time.

You may take several oaths in your life; if you're lucky, they'll never come in conflict with one another. But try looking the mother of your children in the face and telling her that you have no idea why her best friend is so upset. Does it have anything to do with her pregnancy? "Well, yes, sort of. Well, no, not really. Well, I really can't say. What I mean is this: I have no idea!"

You find yourself lying to the one person in the world to whom you swore you would never lie. And yet you also swore that without the patients' permission you would never reveal anything told to you in confidence. Even a dense physician can start to understand the wisdom of never treating one's own family and close friends.

Now, I told her first thing that this test result was probably a false positive. The HIV screen is only that, and many previous viral infections could have caused cross-reacting antibodies. Besides, with her history, she'd had no possible exposure. We'd simply have to wait the ten days (which happened to be the ten days prior to Christmas) for the confirmatory western blot to return totally negative, as it surely would, and then we could ignore the screen results.

The western blot came back positive for every single antibody tested. In fact, it even carried a statement which read, "This patient has been exposed to the HIV virus and should be considered actively infected." It didn't read "might" or "could" have been exposed. It said she *had been exposed.*

Shocked is not adequate to describe my feelings. I called the lab and got verbal confirmation of the written result I had already received by fax. Now what was I going to do? How do I tell her this at ten weeks of pregnancy? How do I tell her there's a 50% chance her baby will be infected? How do I casually work into the conversation the fact that her husband and six-year-old son may already be infected?

I talked to Sharon and her husband in person at my office. I was as gentle as I know how to be, but it was brutal nevertheless. I'm sure they visualized, as I did, the specter of a fetus doomed to die and her son without a mother sometime in the near future. When the tears and sobs abated for a moment, a new story came out.

They were sorry that they'd lied to me, but Kevin was not their own child naturally, at least not her husband's. He had always been sterile, and the boy in fact was conceived by artificial insemination as well; except that seven years before, the donor sperm was fresh, not frozen, and none of the donors were tested for AIDS at that time.

This little bit of information qualified as a bombshell. While the western blot is considered definitive, I sent both their samples to another lab for independent confirmation. This was only a formality, since I had never heard of a 100% positive western blot being in error unless the wrong person's blood was tested. I extracted the appropriate information about which doctors had helped her in the past and learned that two had treated her using the sperm of eight donors in all.

Immediately, we began the time-intensive task of tracking down all the donors by phone. Only one was still in Texas. The other seven lived all over the United States, Canada, and Europe. Unfortunately, before even beginning the search, I knew what the results would be. Without a doubt, my wife's best friend would die young.

Miraculously, after about a week, we had tracked down all but one donor. All were healthy, and all had HIV tests negative within the last year. The final donor was in the USAF, assigned to the Aleutians. It took to the last minute of nine days to get the clearance to confirm that he too was healthy and had tested negative on his recent HIV test.

So, was there some more history lurking here? Unfortunately, I had to approach that directly with Sharon, who was of course offended. No, neither she nor her husband were involved with any drugs or deviant sexual practices. Now my wife's best friend was more upset than ever, and the pressure from my wife was becoming unbearable.

The following day, the day after Christmas that particular year, the second laboratory's results on Sharon and her husband came back. Not only was their western blot totally *negative*, but even their screens were negative!

I was flabbergasted. I had brought this woman almost to the brink of suicide, according to both her and her husband's accounts. I had waited for the supposedly foolproof confirmatory test before even discussing the need for further testing of her husband and son. For a little while at least, I had devastated a family.

After being flabbergasted, I was furious. It took almost a week of phone calls to all sorts of people at this national lab before I could get any inkling of an explanation. It turned out that the screening test, although reported as positive or negative, is actually an antibody titer.

If the results are > 1.00 it is reported as positive. Period. No borderlines, no repeats, no maybes. Sharon's result had been 1.09. It turns out that most positives that are true findings have numbers like 4.0 to 20.0. This information, however, was not available to me as the clinician because the lab felt all suspicious screens should receive further testing.

I called the patient and, of course, relayed the good news about the second lab's results. A third lab later independently confirmed the negative results. Finally, in return for this information, I was freed to let my wife in on the events of the last several months. I can clearly recall the weight instantly lifting from my shoulders.

Such questions of confidentiality are a constant in the physician's life, especially given the rather intimate nature of gynecology.

○○○

Another time I was seeing a young woman, thirty-weeks pregnant, on a routine visit. I commented on the bruises liberally distributed across her upper arms, her throat, her breast, and her buttocks.

She started to cry. I asked her directly if her husband did this to her. "Yes," she finally choked out. "He's really gentle, he just flies into a rage when he's drunk and I don't want to make love, or when the baby cries, or when he's having trouble at work. Please don't say anything. He loves me, he really does, but, but, he'd *kill me* if he knew I'd said anything!"

Well, an ordinary problem of confidentiality, you say. Do you report this to the police? Do you call a battered woman's shelter? Can you do any of that when the patient begs you not to?

How about throwing this in the pot? Her husband was the son of a physician with whom I trained for many years and consider to be one of my closest friends. "No," the patient responded when I asked. "My father-in-law knows nothing about this, and he never will!"

I've got an obligation to protect my patient's health. Preventing further battery falls within the scope of that obligation, does it not? Well, not if your intervention is refused, it doesn't.

Oh, I did the usual things. I gave her the information about area shelters. I urged her to dump the "gentle" jerk that day, right then, right that minute. Take your little girl and don't ever go back there. But she went home like most do, convinced that she was trapped. Who knows? She may be lucky. She went on to have the baby and is now pregnant with a third. She tells me he only cuffs her around once every few months now, but then he isn't home much.

The temptation to involve her physician father-in-law is almost overwhelming. I know him to be a decent, caring man, and I would have presumed a good father. Surely he has no idea this is going on or the potential danger in which his grandchildren could find themselves. But what if he *does* know or suspects? No, breaking a confidentiality in any other situation than direct danger to a minor is always the wrong choice. I kept my mouth shut.

ooo

Then there's the thirty-four-year-old North Dallas beauty. Tennis player, Junior League, circle at church, two kids, Chevy Suburban, and now condyloma accuminatum or venereal warts.

"What should I do? Could I tell my husband I got this fifteen years ago?"

"Did you?"

"Well, no," she says with a sheepish grin.

"Do you have another sexual partner currently?"

"Well, I know it sounds too trite, but yes, I've been sleeping with the tennis pro at the club. Couldn't you just treat me, and then if it comes up talk with my husband and tell him it's been dormant for years?"

While this seems a little more heinous than writing a note to the airline documenting the illness for which the patient tells you she missed her flight, despite the fact that she never contacted your office at the time, the principle is the same. Lying about something and keeping something confidential are two different things. I refused the debutante's request but did tell her our conversation would remain sacrosanct. If her husband should query me, he would be directed to discuss the matter further with his wife.

Yesterday a Middle Eastern patient of mine presented to the office for placement of an IUD. We discussed risks and benefits at length, and realizing that after four children at age thirty, she was perhaps an optimum candidate, I agreed to place the IUD.

After the placement, during the vaginal ultrasound to confirm proper positioning, she mentioned casually that, by the way, if her husband knew about this, he would slit her throat! (Excuse me, *whose* throat did you say he would slit?) Presto change-o, a routine contraceptive visit just became an issue of confidentiality. No billing statements saying "IUD." Questions: will he be able to feel the string? Will this last until menopause? Can it fail? Will it show up on an X-ray? Will it set off the metal detectors at the airport?

# Disrobe Completely

An attractive forty-year-old patient desperately wants to be pregnant. She claims to have been unsuccessful at conceiving despite using no birth control during her three-year marriage. Her husband, a pilot, never comes with her to any visits. She says it's his schedule. She convinces me that he is unwilling to do the usual semen analysis; besides, why would it be needed? He's fathered two children in his previous marriage.

Well, why indeed? Her work-up proceeds. She starts on fertility pills to help her ovulate. Despite success with induction of ovulation over the course of several months, she fails to conceive. We perform an HSG, the X-ray to see if her tubes are patent. As often occurs, there is some therapeutic benefit, and the patient becomes pregnant the next month. Then the phone call.

"Dr. Thurston?"

"Yes, what can I do for you? And by the way, congratulations!"

"That's what I wanted to talk about. You need to know that I don't want you to mention anything about the infertility at our first obstetric appointment. Is that a problem?"

"Not a problem, but do you mind telling me why not?"

"Well, Harry never wanted to have any more children. He sort of doesn't know about my visits for the last six months."

"Sort of?"

"He thinks I get a lot of yeast infections. So, mum's the word, OK?"

I gave her the short course on, "Oh, what a tangled web we weave, when first we practice to deceive," but I think it was lost on her.

○○○

It's Friday afternoon at 4:50 p.m. I am not on call Friday night, nor any night that weekend. Ahhhhhh. But wait, I have forgotten what I do for a living and the power of the hex mentioned earlier. No one else has to mention that when you're not on call; you only have to *think it* for the obstetric gods to get you.

# Sacred Trust

My nurse knocks on the frame of the open door to my office.

"Sorry about this, but Keesha just called, and she says she's started bleeding and is having terrible pelvic pain. I told her to come on in."

"You did the right thing. She only had her surgery two weeks ago, and who knows what might be going on."

Keesha had had a vaginal hysterectomy for heavy bleeding and fibroids. She's done well after the surgery, but I knew she was athletic, active, the mother of three teenagers and had a full-time job; if anyone was going to overdo it, it was Keesha.

My nurse checked her in quickly about twenty minutes later. One of the receptionists up front was staying late for the paperwork, and of course, Evelyn, my nurse, was staying as well. I asked Evelyn what was going on before I took the chart off the outside of the door, and she indicated the patient was obviously upset and in pain, but it wasn't clear just what was happening.

We both entered the room. The patient was sitting on the end of the exam table, a paper sheet across her lap, having been instructed to disrobe from the waist down. She was obviously apprehensive and in not a little bit of pain. I pulled up the stool and positioned her legs as usual in the stirrups, reassuring her all along that it was probably something minor. I did note a trickle of blood from the vagina even before inserting the speculum.

Now, despite years of training and a fair acquisition of that *aequanimitas* thing we alluded to in an earlier chapter, it's hard to contain your surprise when you find things, well, in the wrong place. In this case, for instance, immediately after inserting the speculum I was greeted by a small amount of blood and a large amount of small intestines. I don't think you have to have completed an Ob/Gyn residency to recognize immediately that something was pretty seriously wrong here.

"Keesha, ah, we have a bit of a problem here." I tried to sound nonchalant but am pretty sure I failed miserably. "The kind of problem that will require us taking you across the street to the operating room and doing a little stitching while you take a brief nap."

"What do you mean? What's wrong?" There was just a touch of panic in her voice at this point.

"Well, it seems that the scar at the top of the vagina has separated and your intestines are protruding. You didn't by any chance have sex did you? I mean you knew you couldn't have sex for six weeks, right?"

There was a brief embarrassed silence.

"Well, water under the bridge now." I tried to rescue her. As I headed for the door and Evelyn was helping her up, I told her I would give her husband a call and have him come over right now and take her across the street. When my hand touched the door, Keesha started to sob.

"Wait, doctor. I have to, have to . . . speak with you alone for a moment." I glanced at Evelyn, and she picked up the chart, left the room, and closed the door behind her.

Keesha got herself under control and then looked straight at the floor, as she sat on the side of the bed. "You can't call my husband."

"Excuse me? I can't call your husband?" I am such a dolt sometimes.

"It wasn't him. It wasn't my husband. I'm a flight attendant and I, well, sort of have a boyfriend who's a pilot, and he flew into town last night, and well, I saw him at noon today at his hotel."

"You're kidding me, right?" Sometimes I am just, well, priceless.

"You can't tell him what happened. When you call him, my husband, and tell him to come, you can't tell him what happened. Okay? He has no idea. Believe me, no idea." (I couldn't help thinking, *Nor does anyone else, like your kids, your pastor, your doctor, your neighbor.*)

She looked up at me with tears streaming down her face, and while I had a little trouble feeling sorry for her, I did feel sorry for the human condition in general. What a mess we are!

"No, of course not. I couldn't tell him anything without your permission anyway. We'll just think of something to tell him, that's all."

After I had finished the repair in the operating room, I came out to let her husband know everything had gone well. He made some remark about how that's what I had said after the hysterectomy, and it hadn't gone so well, had it? How could this happen? They hadn't even had sex yet, and still the vaginal cuff had fallen apart! Had I just done sort of a sloppy job the first time?

Whew, talk about drawing on my self-control. No, I said, I'd done the procedure just the same way I had hundreds of times before. I guess sometimes people just don't heal so well.

I left an angry husband, an attorney, who was no doubt thinking of suing.

I could only pray for his sake that it never came to that because some of those depositions, I guarantee, he wouldn't want to hear.

○○○

"Evelyn, how could Jennifer possibly be on the schedule *again*?" After noting that the same young woman had been seen each of the last two months, both times with the same problem.

"Sorry, Doctor T, but I think it might be the same complaint!"

"That is just not possible! If it's right, you better put her in room 3 and plan on not using it again for the rest of the day."

Jennifer, a twenty-two-year-old property manager, unfortunately seemed to have developed a habit of coming in for the same problem repeatedly. About three weeks after each of her last three periods, she had developed a discharge, some irritation, and always a very foul odor.

After Evelyn had her in the designated room undressed from the waist down, I came in with her chart in hand.

# Disrobe Completely

"Okay Jennifer, you don't think, I mean you don't think you forgot . . ."

She looked somewhere between horrified and embarrassed beyond imagination.

"I'm afraid so."

"I am so sorry to sound incredulous, but isn't this the third time in a row? I mean no one wants to be remembered for this, but I believe you've just gone into the record books!"

"I just do not get it! How could I forget again? I mean, this is ridiculous!" She scooted down to the edge of the table, and I helped her into position and then started her exam. "Well, is it?"

When I looked in the speculum, sure enough, there was a retained tampon pushed up into the corner of the vaginal vault called the fornix. I removed the deteriorating cotton wadding with a ring forcep and slipped it quickly into the proffered latex glove which the registered nurse held at arm's length, so that the offensive item could be immediately entrapped, sealed, and then put into the hinged hazardous waste container. As I prepared to wipe the vault clean with a betadine antiseptic solution, incredibly, another tampon became visible. After it, too, was removed and the clean-up completed, the patient hastily returned to the sitting position with her hands over her face.

"This just isn't possible. I mean, I've made love with my husband at least three times since my last period. Does that mean those things were . . ."

"Afraid so," I answered with a bit of a little smile but also a touch of regurgitation in the back of my throat. "I am so sorry Jennifer, but you simply have to tell me what you're doing."

"What do you mean?" she said, looking up with her arms now clasped tightly around her own upper body.

"I mean, tell me what you do from start to finish."

"Well, just what I've always done, I mean, I open the box, take out a tampon, strip off the wrapper, cut off the string and then . . ."

"Whoa! HOLD UP! Stop right there!! You do what?"

"I cut off the string?" she answered questioningly. "Is that a problem?"

"Well, I'd go way out on a limb here and say, YES! Why do you think they put a string on there in the first place? Why on earth do you cut it off?"

She seemed surprised I would even ask. "Well, I don't want to tee-tee on it!"

Okay, I admit it, I'm a guy, even if I am a gynecologist, but I am absolutely positive there are other ways to handle this situation. I discussed with her the options of simply removing the tampon and replacing it, or if she preferred, even holding the string out of the way. Remarkably, she had never used either of these approaches. After a brief revisiting of the toxic shock scares in the eighties and nineties, Jennifer was able to see that perhaps my approach might be better. We left it on a light note, and I swore that this little episode would never leave the room. She's two babies down the line, and I can report that it has yet to leave that room . . . well, except for this book, but since I am *sure* she's never told anybody about it, we should be safe.

$$\bigcirc\bigcirc\bigcirc$$

So confidentiality protects the victimized, the guilty, and the just flat-out embarrassed. It solidifies a relationship that may leave the physician in an uncomfortable position but ensures that the patient can trust her doctor with things that no one else is allowed to know.

There's an obvious practical benefit to this trust. Once patients learn that they can trust you completely, they will be more likely to reveal factors that lead to accurate diagnosis and treatment. For example, if a patient can tell you that, yes, she and her partner practice oral sex, and, yes, he sometimes gets fever blisters, then the diagnosis of genital herpes can remain in the embarrassing category and not move into the suspicion-of-infidelity category that would otherwise result. Confidentiality can thus avoid a potentially catastrophic result for those involved.

Good doctors can be relied upon to be good secret keepers. Even if keeping some secrets is painful or seems ethically wrong at the time or just plain difficult because the secret is so darn funny, its value to the physician-patient relationship is incalculable.

# Shell Shocked

*Physicians tend to dwell more on their failures than their successes. I am sure this is related to their type-A, obsessive-compulsive personality profile. If a patient dies or has serious complications or even if she just doesn't get what she came to me for in the first place, I can agonize over it for weeks, months, or sometimes years, driving those around me to distraction.*

*"What about the six thousand happy, healthy bundles of joy you've helped bring into the world?" my nurse might ask. "Think about them now and then!" She is right, of course, a given in our relationship. So much is right about this world—from the flowers to the ocean, to the mountains, to first love, to everlasting love, to the innocence of a five-year-old. We should focus on that from time to time and not dwell on what's wrong in the world.*

*My job as an obstetrician allows me a very special part in the joy of so many that the anguish of a few should not overshadow it. Recently, I had a photograph taken with a woman and her five children, all of whom I delivered. As a part of her family, I can't help but care what happens to her in a very genuine way. There is something intangible but vital in that—something that must not be lost.*

A few minutes ago I helped ease out her little head, unwrapped the umbilical cord from around her neck, and then slapped her vigorously on the chest after her mother pushed her the rest of the way into the world. There was no sound for a moment, as dad looked through the viewfinder of his video camera, as mom strained to see between her outstretched legs, as the nurse and anesthetist considered their next move if needed, and as I clamped and cut the cord.

When I swung the baby rapidly from upside down to right side up, she did what almost all babies do to greet the new world—she screamed. Mom started crying quietly and dad yelled, "It's a girl, honey, it's a girl!" The nurse spread the baby blanket across the patient's chest, and I gently laid the still wailing, squirming, slippery newborn in her mother's arms.

If you've had a healthy baby, you understand. But unless you're a nurse, midwife, or obstetrician, you've not been able to experience the miracle of new life more than a few times at most. For those of us who have seen it thousands of times, it never loses any of its novelty.

Birth is without a doubt the strongest evidence on earth for the existence of God. There are very few atheist parents. Those that exist must consciously work to avoid the obvious. It's on their newborn's face as she sleeps. It's on his face when he takes his first steps. It's written all over the smile of accomplishment for simply peeing in the potty. It's there when your kids scream, "It's Daddy! He's home!"

My history with Martha went back eight years to a Sunday morning at 3:00 a.m. (I am *not* kidding), when I had operated on her for a ruptured tubal ectopic pregnancy. Two years later, I had delivered her first child—a close call I'll never forget.

Martha had delivered vaginally with no problem. The baby was resting comfortably over in the warmer. But after the delivery of the placenta, she continued to bleed. Her uterus was intermittently boggy, or atonic, and its failure to contract after a long, hard labor was allowing her continued hemorrhage. IV pitocin, im methergine, im prostaglandin f2alpha were all instituted.

# Shell Shocked

The joy of having kept her on the planet two years before was slipping from my hands as she bled profusely despite my best efforts. Her terrified husband was escorted from the room as I explained to Martha, who had no epidural, that we would have to put her to sleep to explore the uterus.

After she was out, we ordered four units of blood typed and crossed, and I told the nurse that I was going to need help retracting to see adequately in the apex of the vagina. She called out of the room for any doctor to come help STAT in room 24.

Two physicians came immediately. They weren't my partners. They weren't close friends. In this time of litigious wildfire, they didn't have to come at all. But they did.

With better lighting and exposure, I could see that the patient had a vaginal sidewall tear that extended all the way up into the cervix and out of sight into the lower part of the uterus. This had occurred spontaneously—no forceps, no vacuum. It was rare but there, nonetheless. Her uterus began to firm up under the combined effects of the medications and continued massage, but the flow of blood continued.

She received those four units. And with the help of the other docs, we repaired her tear. Her recovery was unremarkable. But her gratitude was not. It was expressed in a plaque honoring her daughter's birth and thanking the physicians who saved her life. It was also expressed with a sizable donation to the hospital.

Martha's next delivery was a scheduled cesarean because we were all nervous. The one after that was a vaginal birth after C-section (VBAC) because we were a little less nervous. Even then she had the complication of a retained placenta due to a secondary lobe we were unaware of at delivery. Her final delivery was the one that begins this chapter—perfect.

All of Martha's children are miracles. All of them came long after the ruptured ectopic, which would likely have been fatal less than twenty years ago.

# Disrobe Completely

The first child was delivered only moments before what would surely have been another fatal event, had the delivery not occurred in a modern hospital with skilled physicians in attendance. I will always be a part of this family, and I know that whatever I can do to help them in the future, I will go out of my way to do.

○○○

Sheila was twenty-eight years old at the time. A tiny woman, barely five feet tall, she had labored for twenty-two hours after induction because of toxemia. After pushing for three hours, we were forced to perform a cesarean. The baby was healthy. Mom did well. Everyone was happy until about thirty minutes later in the recovery room when her bleeding picked up markedly. She, too, was a victim of atony, or a uterus that failed to stay contracted and thus stem the flow of blood immediately after birth and the subsequent delivery of the placenta.

We returned to the operating room. I hurriedly discussed the situation with her very loving and concerned husband and received the expected instructions to do whatever was necessary. I assured him it would probably be easy to get a handle on. It was not. We tried massage of the uterus directly with the abdomen open; we directly injected it with the same type of medicines we had used systemically; and we tried packing it, all to no avail. Reluctantly, we proceeded with a hysterectomy while we transfused to her the first of what were to be more than eighteen units of blood. Believing her bleeding controlled, we closed after the hysterectomy. I had another talk with her husband, who was looking shell-shocked at this time. His wife had had a narrow escape, and their childbearing days were now over.

We were back ninety minutes later with bleeding from the vaginal cuff and the left pelvic sidewall. (Toxemia or preeclampsia leads to disorders in the coagulation system as well as fragile edematous [swollen] tissues.) After another hour of surgery, we believed all the bleeding was stopped that could be stopped. We left special packs in place and transferred her to the ICU, intubated and unconscious. Fifteen liters of saltwater had made her extremely swollen and pale. I assured the husband once again that I thought we were over the hump.

We were not. One hour later we were back in the OR. I had called in a gynecological oncologist familiar with bleeding dyscrasias (abnormalities) as well as surgery in the deep pelvic sidewall. We worked for another two hours along with one of my partners, now also present at 2:00 a.m. It was all to no avail. We continued to transfuse her and could not stop the bleeding surgically. The tissue was too fragile, and vessels just ripped open when in contact with suture.

I was aware of a relatively new procedure from a conference out in California I had attended just two months before. One of the topics was uncontrollable pelvic sidewall hemorrhage. The procedure described involved embolizing small pieces of foam into larger arteries with a catheter while under flouroscopic guidance in radiology.

Faced with the imminent death of this new mother, we called in the only radiologist in town with experience in the area. We rapidly closed the patient and got her transported—multiple IVs, bladder catheter, endotracheal (breathing) tube, ventilator, and all—to radiology. Over the next hour and a half, a new technology, the devotion of a skilled radiologist, and perseverance saved her life. It was truly a miracle!

Sheila continues to be one of my happiest patients. Always with a smile on her face, she revels in the constant joy of a growing son and, perhaps, in seeing the sun rise each new day.

It was dedicated people in the middle of the night, it was continuing medical education, it was brand new technology that saved her life. I believe dedication, education, and research and development may all be critically wounded by managed care. If that happens, another Sheila in the future will die.

# Disrobe Completely

○○○

I used to be a doctor. I spent my days and nights as I have described above. I know these cases were out of the ordinary, but every day, every physician involved in direct patient care does something that our parents would have deemed miraculous. For example, no matter what you believe the acceptable cesarean-section rate should be, there is no one who argues that in at least 5-10% of deliveries it is lifesaving to mother and child.

What happened before the second decade of this century when the baby was too big for the birth canal? Well, midwives or doctors used instruments to destroy the fetal skull if possible and extract the fetus. If this wasn't possible, then hemorrhage, sepsis, exhaustion, and death for mother and child were inevitable.

How about ectopic pregnancy, until recently the number-one cause of maternal deaths in this country? Now most tubal pregnancies are caught early via radioimmunoassay blood analysis and vaginal ultrasound. We can treat the ectopic laparoscopically (telescope inserted in the navel) with remote-controlled instruments or, more recently, even treat it with chemotherapy and avoid surgery altogether.

Doctors, aided by other paramedical personnel, perform lifesaving miracles every day. But now they tell me I'm a health care provider, not a miracle worker. What on earth are they talking about?

# This Is Embarrassing, But . . .

Something truly wonderful can happen between a patient and her physician. When that special something clicks and you both know it's a good fit, the door opens to all sorts of ways in which the physician and the patient can help each other.

I've learned the value of trying to achieve the necessary sense of trust right from the first interview. It is that sense of trust that allows the discussion of the most intimate details of a patient's life. These very private areas often include those that are causing her the most pain and distress.

I can't believe I'm telling you this . . . I've never even talked out loud about this before." The young woman's voice was shaky as she dabbed at her eyes with the proffered tissue.

"You'll notice I have a box strategically placed in sixteen places in every room."

She laughed as she sat back in her chair and took a deep breath.

"I feel so stupid asking you about this when I hardly know you. I've wanted to talk about it for two years, but no one ever seemed like the right person to listen."

Dana crossed her arms over the purse in her lap, still clutching the wadded tissue. She was a strikingly beautiful, twenty-eight-year-old woman with shoulder-length, dark-brown hair and penetrating hazel eyes. She was "dressed for success" in a forest green suit and understated gold jewelry.

"Don't ever think your questions are stupid," I told her. "They told Ben Franklin, Madame Curie, and Thomas Edison that their questions were stupid, you know. Sex should be fun. It's healthy, it's a normal part of a loving relationship, and if you don't do something about the pain you've been having, it could destroy even the strongest relationship. You know it's no fun making love to a woman in pain. Men may be insensitive jerks a lot of the time, but even the dense ones know when you're having a good time and when you're not. If your husband knows he's hurting you, then he probably feels like an ax murderer every time!"

"Oh, he knows it hurts, but he's so gentle. We've tried everything. Different lubricants, different positions. I've been treated for yeast infections, bacterial infections, had my hormones tested, been off the pill, on the pill . . . nothing seems to help." Dana started to cry again, and I freshened her tissue from the box on the desk next to the picture of my kids and my dog.

"Now we don't make love at all. He's good about it, but, well, he's frustrated." I could hear the frustration in her voice as well.

"You may have noticed a fundamental principle of nature through all this, not applicable in every case of course, but still a good generalization," I said.

"What's that?" She looked up from her lap to me.

"Why, that men are horny 100% of the time! Believe it or not, it really is the male 'love language' most of the time. Not service. Not quality time. The old adage is true, 'Men need sex to be close. Women need to be close to have sex.' No matter how much he loves you, especially if you had the good sexual relationship that you described for the first two years, this problem will erode other aspects of your life together. So, we'll just have to fix it."

We spent the next thirty minutes during that first interview talking about possible causes for sudden onset of severe pain on insertion after years of having no problem whatsoever with the same partner. Sometimes all it takes is intercourse during a severe yeast infection or a brief period of inadequately lubricated intercourse to develop a reflex tightening of the strong muscles around the opening of the vagina. This is called vaginismus. It is not under the patient's conscious control any more than the knee-jerk reflex.

We discussed the use of vaginal stents or dilators of successively larger diameter held in place each night for fifteen to twenty minutes. If done over six weeks, during which time the patient is abstinent, this can completely cure the problem. We discussed other conditions more difficult to treat, such as vestibular adenitis, a viral infection of the tiny glands that surround the opening of the vagina or vestibule. The infection could be acquired sexually and then rapidly lead to the scenario wherein penetration was no longer tolerable. Its treatment would involve new concepts such as serial injection with interferon and possibly surgical reconstruction.

Dana left the first interview with new hope. True, she had to suffer through the brief biography I give to all new patients, supplemented by diplomas and my kids' pictures around the office, the Christian Medical and Dental Society plaque over my credenza, and the Bible on the desk, but I think openness about your own life and experiences fosters openness in the patient.

Dana and I started down a long road together that day. The sequential dilators failed. A laparoscopy did not reveal endometriosis or any other underlying cause for previous deep pain that could have led to pain at the introitus (opening). Painful sequential interferon injections, three times per week over four weeks, failed to relieve her pain, although they work 70% of the time. She almost lost her fiancé at that point. Finally, four months after she started seeing me, we agreed to surgical excision of the effected area. She was scared and so was I. The surgery can leave scarring that could worsen things, if that were possible.

But it didn't. Her pain resolved completely when she resumed intercourse six weeks after surgery. She and her fiancé got married, and I have since delivered a boy and a girl to the happy couple.

# Disrobe Completely

Restoring a young woman's sexuality is quite simply a wonderfully gratifying thing. It is, in a very real sense, saving a life as much as operating on an ectopic pregnancy or performing an emergent cesarean section. Since my first successes at it, I have learned to probe for problems in this area of life that many patients are at first reticent to discuss. They're embarrassed and often think the problem is unique to them. Asking about it frankly reassures them that many people suffer from the same problems often brings on a torrent of tears, but they're tears of relief.

Gynecologists do have a unique perspective on the doctor-patient relationship. Over 90% of health problems in women under age fifty involve their reproductive system (both organs and hormones) or their breasts. Thus the very nature of our interaction with the patient is intimate, even without a word spoken. People are taught from age two that their genitals are their "privates," and most of them take it to heart.

But sexuality is not the only intimacy with which we deal. Women face problems with bowel and bladder function, infertility, weight loss, hair loss, mood swings, depression, bloating, breast tenderness, menstrual pain and/or heavy flow, and incredible stress with the triple role of wife, mom, and business executive. And unfortunately, in our society, women also face the problem of battery and sexual abuse.

Sensitivity to these issues derives from a trusting physician-patient relationship that cannot be quantified. While some patients may tell me their intimate sexual problems at a first meeting (my mom says that I just have the kind of face that invites people to pour stuff out), most save those discussions until they feel certain that I am empathetic and can be trusted with a confidence. Often this comes after the delivery of a child. If you share what is arguably the most significant single event in a woman's life (and you're not a schmuck), she then lets you into a part of her that is reserved for very few. This intimacy provides an opportunity to offer help in ways that no stranger could.

# This Is Embarrassing, But . . .

Knowledge of her relationship with her spouse and her children allows the physician to make the treatment decisions best suited to her life. This may be manifested in as simple an issue as choosing the right method of birth control or as complicated an issue as how to best approach her depression.

All of you men reading this will understand one manifestation of this relationship. Try getting your wife to leave a gynecologist with whom she's comfortable because your company offers a PPO that doesn't include her doctor. It may seem irrational to you that she's willing to pay more per month to continue with her old doctor, but perhaps a woman places a different value than a man on having found someone with whom she can talk comfortably.

When I was a doctor, a trusting relationship was central to my successful interaction with every patient possible. As a health care provider with annual patient exchange due to shifting contracts, limitations imposed by insurers on my authority to make the right decisions, frustration and time wasted on paperwork and the phone, and an ever-worsening liability crisis, I wonder if I will be caring for the patients with the same concern and compassion that I once could. You can decide for yourself after reading part 3.

"To paint a fine picture is far more important than to sell it."

—Edward Alden Jewell

# Part 3

# Have a Seat on the Table:

## Reality

*There was a time not so very long ago when you could walk into any surgeon's lounge in the country and really learn something about medicine. As a resident in the early eighties, I remember rotating to the private hospitals in the Bay Area and learning as much or more in the lounge as I did in the operating room.*

*The reason was simple. Medicine was exciting. It was fun. People enjoyed what they did for a living, and they liked to talk about it. We knew our patients and cared deeply about new ways to help them. The potential benefits of a new procedure would be touted by one doctor and shot down by another. One doctor would have closed this way, and another, in a completely different way. Doctor X swore by this type of suture, and another physician knew it was worthless for all the following reasons. Under normal circumstances, two doctors will debate about almost anything to do with medicine. Marshalling your arguments and championing the procedures that you feel hold the most merit is the process of medical education.*

*Walk into a surgeon's lounge today, and you'll hear only two basic topics being discussed: managed care/health care-reform and medical-legal issues. That's it. Period. I guarantee it. Outside of consultations, I haven't heard an honest discussion about how best to approach a patient's problem for probably ten years.*

*Today, the frustration born of outside interference with diagnostic and treatment decision-making is so overwhelming that it occupies physicians almost to the exclusion of any other topics—with the exception of lawsuits. Medical-legal concerns are omnipresent, at least for those in my specialty. The American College of Obstetricians and Gynecologists' survey in 1990 first revealed that 77.6% of all Ob/Gyn physicians had been sued; the average number of claims filed against them was 2.5. The numbers are no better today. An ACOG news release in 2000 revealed that the average Ob/Gyn would be sued 2.53 times in his career. There is a 90% chance that an Ob/Gyn will be sued at least once in his lifetime, so there's an excellent chance that several of the physicians in that lounge at any given moment are involved in the endless grind of ongoing litigation.*

*So the talk is of HMOs, PPOs, co-pays, pre-certification, quality assurance, value enhancement, capitation, de-selection, Congress, HIPAA, JCAH, pre-existing conditions, etc. We moan and gnash our teeth about malpractice premiums, letters of intent, depositions, expert witnesses, plaintiffs with spurious complaints, outrageous jury decisions and phenomenal awards, and losing our patients if insurance companies de-select us as providers, or their employers change plans. We swap horror stories of doctors facing financial ruin and despair. We share our fears about loss of retirement funds and the disruption of our children's education.*

*But there is no talk about medicine. None. There is no talk of the patients. Where is the compassion now? There is only concern with the self. And there is fear—fear so real you can smell it. I believe this to be a symptom of a very serious disease with a dismal prognosis unless we intervene immediately and forcefully. Doctors are becoming health care providers by default. Our time, our efforts, our concentration, our energy, and our emotions are being drained by these issues, which do not have direct bearing on the improvement of our ability to care for the patient.*

*The following stories will give you a glimpse of the way in which managed care coupled with a lack of tort reform is unraveling our system by inexorably destroying what we once knew as the physician and replacing him with a "provider."*

# Patient Name and Group Number

*As the decision-making power of your physician is stripped away, he is left powerless to do the right thing for your health. This alarming trend may have started with a little hesitation on the part of insurers to pay for 80% of everything with carte blanche, but it has escalated to the point where poor decisions about your health are made by uninformed individuals solely on the basis of cost. That means mounting frustration for doctors. And that, as we shall see, leads rapidly to danger for patients.*

P lease continue holding. Your call is important to us. Do not hang up. Your call will be answered in the order in which it is received . . ."

I think I'd rather hear this disembodied, computer-generated voice over and over than return to the inevitable piano solo of "Feelings." But since the average time on hold can range from as little as two minutes to as long as forty minutes, there is usually ample opportunity to listen to both.

There was a time, they tell me, when a physician never had to speak to an insurance company representative on the phone. In fact, there was a time when the physician's office rarely spoke with an insurance company. It's not that there is anything particularly distasteful about speaking on the telephone. It is, however, difficult to do so for every single procedure, surgery, hospital admission, hospital stay, etc.

This time, after only seventeen minutes, a different voice comes over the speakerphone on the credenza behind my chair. I whirl around, snatching the handset from the cradle in time to hear . . .

"If you wish to inquire about a specific claim and you are a client, press the pound sign and one NOW. If you are inquiring about your premium or other account information, press the pound sign and two NOW. If you know the party's extension to which you wish to speak, press the pound sign and three NOW. If you are a physician, physician's office, hospital, imaging or surgery center, press the pound sign and four NOW. If you wish to continue holding, please press five, [God's honest truth—press five if I wish to continue holding] hold the line [again], and an operator will [may or may not] be with you soon. . . ."

Like the puppet that I am becoming, I press the pound sign and four.

"You have accessed the health care provider client representative. If you wish to inquire about pre-certification for a procedure or admission, please press one NOW. If you wish to obtain a referral code number, press two NOW. If you wish to discuss reimbursement on a claim already filed, please press three NOW. If you need further assistance, please stay on the line and an operator will be with you soon."

I press one and pray that I'm almost out of the loop. After all, I do have three patients in the exam rooms. Since I'm scheduled in surgery during the insurer's lunch hour and their closing time is 5:00 p.m. EST, I must call between patients.

"Good afternoon, APSCO Insurance. 'Your Health Is Our Concern.' Angela speaking. How may I help you?" Well, this is a start.

"This is Dr. Thurston in Dallas, and I'm calling . . ."

"Do you have the party's name to which you wish to speak?"

"No, I do not. As I was saying, this is Dr. Thurston and . . ."

"Patient name and group number please."

"The patient's name is Jackson, Brooke T., and I don't have the group number. Look I just need to speak to . . ."

"Hold, please," she commands, and I'm back to "Feelings" again.

Now, often this is where I get off. Patients are waiting. Some frontline person has already denied precertification for a medically necessary procedure, and I need to speak to the medical director. But this time I just can't hang up. The procedure is scheduled in two days. The patient informs me she was precertified with no problem; she even had a confirmation number. My office staff was told the opposite on the same day. Dammit, I have to speak to somebody.

"I'm sorry, Doctor, but we have no Brooke D. Jackson. The group number would really help."

"It's T., Brooke T. Jackson, and I'm sure the group number would help, but that doesn't change the fact that I don't have it. Now all I need is . . ."

"No need to get testy now. Hold, please."

It's a good thing not everyone has video phones yet. When they do, I'm going to stop using the telephone completely. After fifteen seconds or so of a refreshing version of "People," Angela returns.

"I have it on screen now, Doctor. How can I help you?"

After an all-too-audible sigh, I try again. "I need to speak to the medical director regarding the denied precertification on Ms. Jackson's laparoscopic ligamentopexy. The patient claims she was precertified; our office was informed that she was not."

"Well, let's see here. Nope. No record of either your office or the patient contacting us about this matter."

My intercom rings. It's my nurse: I've been on the line twenty minutes since the last patient checked out. Mrs. Schwartz is a postpartum and has her pediatrician's appointment in fifteen minutes all the way across town. Candy's crying in the treatment room with that right-side pain again. And Mrs . . .

"I'll be there as soon as I can."

"I'm in Hartford, sir."

"Oh, sorry, not you, that was the intercom. I've ah, ah, got people wait-ing. Look, I know the patient called. She was given a confirmation number. Here, it's on her chart. AP93-117493-22-018."

"Hold, please." Shit! Why does this surprise me every time? Even a fully orchestrated "To Sir, With Love" does little to placate me. After forty-five sec-onds or so, my misnamed Angel returns with good news and bad.

"Dr. Thornton?"

"It's Thurston, Dr. Thurston."

"Well, Dr. Thurston, we do show a Mrs. Jackson receiving that number to precertify a laparoscopic tubal ligation, but after further review and recogniz-ing that her PPO policy does not cover birth control, we informed your office of the reversal and subsequent denial of her precertification."

"That would be just fine, except the procedure requested is a laparoscopic ligamentopexy for chronic dyspareunia."

"This procedure is for ICD9 623.8?"

"Could be, if that's the number for dyspareunia!"

"Well, treatment for painful sex is hardly a medical necessity, now is it?"

"I guess that would depend on your point of view. I would like to speak to the medical director, please."

"Have you tried lubricants? The computer under ICD9 623.9 lists dryness as the most common cause, you know."

"Ma'am, to be honest with you, I don't have the time or the inclination to discuss this with you. Now what is the medical director's name?"

"We don't give out our medical directors' names."

"Well, could you connect me with him now?"

"I'm sorry, that's quite impossible. We will give him the case number and ask him to call you back ASAP."

"Well, might that be this afternoon?" I queried hopefully.

"Most likely tomorrow. Our doctors are very busy, you know."

I wanted to say, "Is that so? Well, I have nothing to do but sit around and play this #@%$%^&*%^ game all day long!" But I just gave her the number for the OB office where I could be reached the following day.

Now, recognizing how difficult it was to make it this far, when a nurse retrieved me from an examining room the following afternoon for the medical director at APSCO's call, I rushed from the patient's room as though it were Ed McMahon at Publishers Clearing House on the line.

"Yeah, this is Dr. Thurston."

"Hello, I understand there is some confusion over Brooke Jackson's precertification?"

"Excuse me, but are you the medical director?" He sounded more like my great-grandfather.

"Yes, that's right, son." *Son*? Can you believe it? He actually called me son. I wanted to address him as Dad, but thought better of it at the last second.

"Your name, please?"

"I am the medical director for this claim. My name is of no consequence. Now how can I help you, Doctor?" The emphasis on the last word established firmly what I had initially suspected. This guy was condescending to me, not vice versa! But if I was ever going to help my patient, I had to continue playing the game.

"My patient has suffered from deep dyspareunia for all of her adult sexual life. She has a severely retroverted, retroflexed uterus, and I believe deep penetration leads to contact with an entrapped ovary."

"Is that ICD9 623.8 or .9?"

Exasperated, I replied through clenched teeth. "I've been told it's 623.9. Does that help?"

"Hold on for a moment, please." Then came "Feelings" again. I was getting nauseous. I think this jerk was actually looking it up on the computer.

"Sorry about that. Listen; have you tried lubricants?"

"You cannot be serious. We have tried everything over the three years that she has been my patient. Her husband is cooperative but as frustrated as she is. It is beginning to seriously tax what is otherwise an apparently loving relationship."

"Well, what is it exactly, that you propose to do?"

"As I said, a laparoscopic ligamentopexy."

"What is that?"

"What is what?"

"A laparoscopic liga . . . whatever you said."

"You're going to decide what procedure is medically necessary, and you don't know what the procedure is?"

"Now you listen to me, son. I was a general practitioner for fifty-five years in Flatbush, Nevada, and believe you me, I've done plenty of procedures, and many I'm sure before you were born, so don't talk down to me, Doctor!"

Stupefied, I actually apologized.

"I'm sorry Doctor . . . er . . . sir, I only find it difficult to understand how you can make a decision in this case."

"Are you going to describe the procedure or not?"

"Yes, sure. It's a laparoscopic procedure wherein the round ligaments are redoubled and thus shortened, pulling the fundus to the anterior abdominal wall with only two small incisions. The ovaries are thus suspended away from the pouch of Douglas."

"Did you say suspended?"

"Yes. So?"

"That's procedure code G421.2. It's not covered. Any uterine suspension is considered elective major surgery and it's not covered. Sorry."

"But that's the point, this procedure doesn't fall under the old code. It's outpatient. It takes maybe thirty minutes and the patient is home in two hours, back to work in three days!"

"Well, there's no code for it specifically. Furthermore, sexual enjoyment hardly seems a life or death matter, does it?"

"I don't think the patient would agree with you. Who else . . ."

"You can't talk to anyone else, Doctor. If Ms. Jackson wants this unnecessary procedure, she can pay for it herself! Good day!"

He hung up! He hung up on me! That was a twist. I usually hang up on "Feelings" or "People" or whatever.

That evening I called Mrs. Jackson and relayed her insurer's opinion. She had exactly no recourse, other than paying legal fees to sue an omnipotent insurance company that could well afford better representation than she. We agreed to talk again soon and try to come up with some other options. But I hung up knowing that the only real option was for her to live with her pain until after she had completed her childbearing, and then pray for some pathology that her insurer would feel qualified her for hysterectomy.

Visualize this type of exchange happening thousands of times every day all over the country. Similar exchanges occur between office personnel and insurance company registered nurses perhaps a hundred times more frequently. Frustration and wasted time are magnified by the fact that insurers use independent agencies on a contract basis to handle precertification. As a consequence, the potential for errors in communication is increased, and the insurer has the opportunity (and frequently uses it) to deny payment retroactively, citing the nonbinding nature of approval before the fact by an outside agency.

In our OB office, we have about nine hundred ongoing pregnancies. Currently, our receptionist has to call for precertification for (1) obstetric care, (2) ultrasound, (3) oral glucose screening for diabetes, (4) vaginal delivery or C-section, (5) hospital admission, and (6) any extension to length of stay. That is about 5,400 more phone calls per year than prior to managed care.

# Disrobe Completely

Each of those phone calls can involve the "please hold" phenomenon for many minutes. Each of those phone calls is an opportunity for human error. Mind you, these 5,400 additional phone calls are for each of the patients with *no* problems. Additional calls are generated for anything out of the routine.

I am confident that any surgeon today could give you examples of the precertification nightmare. One of my colleagues recently carried on a conversation similar to the one I had above. It took over a week before he could actually talk to the medical reviewer for this particular company. After a long discussion about laser endometrial ablation, it became clear to my associate that the reviewer had no idea what he was talking about.

When he repeatedly pressed the reviewer as to her qualifications, she couldn't give an answer to any questions about her internship, residency, practice experience, etc. After several more infuriating phone conversations, my associate discovered that the so-called medical reviewer was in fact a Southern California medical student working on an hourly basis to help defray some of her living expenses. So a *student* made the decision that denied a patient a procedure that my colleague, with twenty years of experience and multiple board certifications, thought was appropriate.

In 1999, I had precertification denied for a repeat cesarean section. I happen to be a relative proponent of VBAC, or vaginal birth after cesarean, in limited circumstances. Educating the patient as to the reasonable safety of trying to deliver vaginally after a previous cesarean did help to lower the repeat section and thus the total C-section rate in the late 1990s. This in turn lowered length of stay, which lowered total cost. (While true in 1999, by 2006 insurance actuarial studies suggested that repeated vaginal delivery increased pelvic support problems later in life, leading to more hysterectomies. This combined with less than reassuring data about the actual risk of VBAC has contributed to the rise of both primary and repeat C-sections across the nation.)

That's all well and good. But VBAC is not appropriate for every clinical situation. The young lady whose precertification was denied had a 16-cm posterior lower uterine segment fibroid (benign uterine tumor) blocking her birth canal. She also had a previous uterine rupture with an attempted VBAC elsewhere. Her insurer *still* denied payment for a scheduled cesarean section!

The patient had a C-section anyway and paid the difference in hospital costs herself. But she was understandably indignant at what she viewed to be potentially dangerous strong-arm tactics to lower the insurer's portion of her hospital costs.

The frustrations are by no means confined to precertification. For the patient with painful intercourse, it is true, the insurance company's decision to deny the procedure may not be life threatening, even if it leads to the dissolution of her marriage. It is also true that the decision with respect to the VBAC patient only cost her money and not her health. But other issues affect the welfare of the patient more immediately. In fact, other managed care rulings on length of stay, choice of pharmaceuticals, choice of laboratory tests, and restriction of appropriate consultation are leading to dangerous situations.

## Outta Here

It has now become commonplace for patients to be discharged at the dictates of the payor without regard to their conditions by people who lack an adequate understanding of the patient's needs.

Classic examples in the obstetric area would include patients seeking admission to the hospital for antepartum care due to high-risk conditions. These commonly include bleeding placenta previa, preterm labor, premature rupture of membranes, and preeclampsia or toxemia.

While it is true that in certain instances all of these situations might be managed with bed rest at home, each individual case is unique.

For instance, a thirty-one week, preterm labor patient on a subcutaneous pump for administration of medicine might have been managed with home monitoring *if* certain conditions were met. Those conditions might include proximity to the hospital, a cervical exam that was not worrisome with respect to dilation, softness, position, effacement, and condition of the lower uterine segment, a vertex presentation, intact membranes, etc.

Let's assume that in this very common, uncomplicated circumstance you have no idea what I am talking about. Now, recognize that we may be seeking approval from an orthopedics nurse on the phone from Hartford, Connecticut, who has no more idea about the subtle difference in situations than you do. She makes the decision about whether the patient can stay in the hospital on the basis of criteria on a computer screen in front of her. Reasoning with her not only can require huge amounts of time but is usually futile. If the patient is not independently wealthy and the screening nurse denies her stay, she's Outta Here.

So let's say the patient lives 120 miles away and has a worrisome cervix but is doing fine at this moment. Does she go home? Of course not, medically. But if her insurance denies her, the hospital wants payment. Even if she chooses to stay and can negotiate with the hospital, the uncovered portion of her bill can be astronomical.

In 1996, I had a patient two days post-C-section with a 102.6-degree fever, a reddening, oozing wound, breast engorgement, and anemia with a blood count of twenty-four (thirty-two is normal post-op). Her insurance refused to pay for continued hospitalization despite IV, antibiotics, lack of bowel function, likely wound infection, and severe anemia with increased pulse and light-headedness.

She left the hospital after two hours of telephone work setting up and approving home care—IVs, nurses, etc. Admittedly, with cost shifting on the hospital's part, each twenty-four hours would run an astonishing $1,800 including nursery care. For home care, the insurer paid only $900 per day. But this patient's care was altered solely on the basis of financial pressure. She was readmitted three days later with a severe postop ileus (lack of bowel function), inability to urinate, continued fever, and a swollen arm from an infiltrated IV. She was in the hospital an additional five days. Was her early discharge either safe or cost-effective? Probably not.

Remarkably, in 1997, with the female former governor of New Jersey leading the charge, the US Congress passed legislation mandating that all insurers must pay for four nights in the hospital after a C-section and two after vaginal delivery. It was one of the most remarkable events in the history of legislative controls over the insurance industry. I am aware of no other single medical procedure for which Congress has mandated insurers cover hospitalization for a specified period of time.

## Not on Our List

Several years ago a patient of mine was diagnosed with a brain tumor of unclear etiology. While imaging studies showed characteristics compatible with a benign meningioma, the neurologist still recommended consultation with a neurosurgeon. The neurosurgeon with whom this neurologist works was not on the patient's PPO list, so he helped her choose one that was.

The approved neurosurgeon agreed that she needed surgery, but when they went to schedule it, they learned the hospital he operated at was not on her PPO list. Appeals to her insurance bureaucracy proved fruitless in the ensuing months. This situation was eventually resolved, but if you were the patient, would you be happy spending three months working with administrative cretins while your brain tumor grew?

This week, a thirty-six-year-old woman and longtime patient of mine presented with gradually worsening left-side pain. The ultrasound in the office revealed that she had a cystic and solid 11-cm ovarian mass. I had delivered all three of her children. I had helped her through the tough times five years before when her mother had died of ovarian cancer. Now she needed me. She needed surgery, but I also think she needed me.

When we started to schedule her surgery, we discovered that she had been seeing me out of network for the last two years and paying out of her pocket for office-visits. I told her I would do the surgery, and she could pay whatever she thought was fair over whatever time she needed.

That didn't solve the problem. The hospital I practice at was no longer on her network. Out-of-network payment to facility in this case was zero. Hospital costs would probably top ten to twelve thousand dollars. She and her firefighter husband just couldn't do it. So with a newly diagnosed tumor and a history of her mother dying of ovarian cancer, she was forced to see a physician she had never seen before at another hospital to have a major surgery performed.

## Not Necessary

Susan had just experienced her fourth consecutive miscarriage. Blood testing of anticardiolipin, lupus anticoagulant, and antinuclear antibody were all negative, as were X-rays of her uterine lining (HSG). Every text in the world agreed that it was time for chromosomal testing of her and her husband. The karyotype on their blood samples would be $310 apiece. Her carrier decided, after multiple discussions with all my office personnel and finally after my discussion with the medical director, that this testing was unjustified. No appeal.

Corazon is a forty-two-year-old Latina patient with a history of tubal ligation. She has periods lasting from fifteen to forty days at a time, which are unresponsive to hormonal treatment due to multiple small uterine fibroids, at least some of which are encroaching on her uterine lining. Her blood count hovers around twenty-five (normal is forty). She has bladder pressure and cramping almost daily. She was scheduled for a total abdominal hysterectomy. Her managed care company said she would need a second opinion. I always welcome second opinions but felt it absurd in this case and expressed this to the nurse reviewer. She said she would present it to the review board and let me know in two days.

True to her word, she called back in two days and told my nurse that a second opinion would not be necessary. Unfortunately, the reason was that they were denying the surgery out of hand. Had I tried hormonal therapy? We reviewed that with them again. Had I considered endometrial ablation? We explained why that was inappropriate. Had the patient ever needed blood transfusion? Well, not yet. We were instructed that when that was the case, her circumstances would be reviewed again. Bye. End of story.

## Denied . . . Preexisting

Let's discuss one of my personal favorite categories. As you are well aware, insurers, whether for life or health, frequently deny applicants coverage on the basis of preexisting conditions. This obviously applies to patients with chronic conditions whether that be arthritis, lupus, psoriasis, etc. With respect to life-insurance coverage, it is logical that a company would not want to pick up someone who already had leukemia, AIDS, lung cancer, or some other definitively terminal process.

But these conditions are not the ones that most frequently lead to a denial of insurance coverage. In fact, many of the conditions that lead to insurance denial, the patient may not even have! Let me clarify this.

Recently a patient of mine was denied life insurance because in her chart, three years and two children before, there was a note about the patient inquiring after the safety of a certain antidepressant while having unprotected sex.

# Disrobe Completely

She was told there would be no problem. Now, she and her husband have applied for life insurance and been denied on the basis of that note. Well, the patient not only was not depressed, but also never took the medicine. She had asked the question for her next-door neighbor! I had never prescribed the drug to her, there was no evidence that she ever took it, yet after multiple communiques and documentation, the insurer would not reconsider.

Another common one for health-insurance is genital herpes or HSV. It is estimated that 67 million Americans have this viral infection (NIAID's STD Fact Sheet, July 1999). We know it is not a precursor to cervical cancer as was once thought; human papilloma virus (HPV) has been identified as the actual guilty virus in this regard. HSV has no long-term health effects. It may not even be necessary to do cesareans for active lesions in the near future, as we have come to realize that only first-time lesions in the last couple weeks of pregnancy hold significant risk for the newborn. Despite these facts, I constantly receive notification that a woman's health-insurance with a new carrier has either excluded coverage for *any* problems with her reproductive tract or denied her coverage completely, solely on the basis of a history of genital herpes.

Now here's the real kicker. I have patients for whom we have suspected genital herpes, cultured for it, had it return negative, never have another suspicious episode, and *still* be denied! I have patients with recurrent abnormal Pap smears for whom we have performed a loop electrosurgical excision (LEEP), removed the worrisome tissue in question, had pathology confirm the absence of true dysplasia or precancerous change under the microscope and had DNA probes prove the absence of the HPV virus, and *still* they are denied coverage in the future.

Preexisting conditions have become a convenient, often undocumented mechanism for insurers to deny coverage of entire portions of a person's health care, like their reproductive tract. Whether it's HSV and denial of maternity benefits or fibrocystic breast changes and subsequent denial of coverage for a totally unrelated breast cancer, current *carte blanche* with respect to the insurer's ability to deny coverage prospectively, as well as retrospectively, adds significantly to the frustrations of health care for both the physician and the patient.

In August of 2006, I walked into the surgeons' lounge to hear one of my colleagues relating another incredible insurance interaction that will strike a chord with any reader who has ever dealt with a medical insurer.

It seemed that my associate Jim's twenty-five-year-old son required the services of a gastroenterologist. Helpful dad that he is, Jim arranged for an appointment to see a GI doc at our institution the next time his son was in Dallas. The evaluation took place at the appointed time, but the history required an additional meeting for an office endoscopy in which the young man was sedated and then required to swallow a flexible fiber-optic telescope. Photos were taken, and after more significant diseases were ruled out, my friend's son was treated for reflux esophagitis, known now as GERD or gastro-esophogeal reflux disease to the millions out there who use Protonix or Nexium or Prilosec.

All was well until Jim received a notification simply stating that his son's workup and treatment would not be covered by his PPO policy (for which I just happen to know he pays roughly $1,100 per month with a $3,000 deductible per person). After playing the hold–push button game you found in the opening pages of the book on the phone with the insurer, he was told that his son was no longer covered because he had turned twenty-five six months prior to his appointment. Well, Jim knew of the insurance company's policy to stop coverage of children over the age of twenty-five. He simply hadn't thought about it at the time of his son's treatment, assuming that as the insurance company managed to send him a statement for premiums each month, they might also have been able to mention in one of those statements that this change in coverage was fast approaching or would happen this month or had recently occurred. But no such notification came from the insurer.

Now, my associate is a reasonable guy. He told the disembodied voice on the phone that he understood. He then inquired how long it would take them to process the reimbursement check for that $200-per-month premium that he had paid over the last six months for a policy the evidently didn't exist. The anonymous insurance company associate—whose first priority is ensuring customer satisfaction—said something along the lines of, "Come again?" Jim explained the logic of his inquiry and was met with a long wait on hold only to be eventually cut off. When he called back, he, of course, got another disembodied voice whose only concern was how she might help him but who naturally required hearing the story from the beginning, including all the necessary numbers to call up the account on the computer screen.

"I'm sorry, sir. But we do not refund premiums." Say what? Premiums for what? Doesn't the term *premium* refer to payment for existing insurance coverage?

"Well," my associate responded, "I guess I need to speak to your supervisor."

"That won't do you any good," was her terse reply. Knowing that was probably true, the good doctor persisted. After another interminable wait, softened only by the theme to *Titanic* (always appropriate), the supervisor came on the line. Need I say that the identification game had to be repeated in its entirety, including the nature of the problem?

"Well, I understand what you're saying Mr. Richards [let's not stand on titles that took nine years after college to acquire], but it is the insured's responsibility to be familiar with the parameters of the policy in question," spoke the supervisor with the tone of a middle-aged schoolmarm, somewhat exasperated by the mental deficiency of the bumpkin on the other end. The doctor/client had grown a tad exasperated at this point, and my partner is a very patient man.

# Patient Name and Group Number

"I understand my responsibility, ma'am. I pay for a product, and you deliver. If I pay for a product in error, one which you are not actually selling, then it stands to reason that you would refund my money in good faith."

"I'm so sorry, sir. [I feel your pain!] But we don't refund premiums."

I have to stop here before I get upset myself. You know what the rest of this scratched record sounds like—an endless cycle of the same nonsensical response. As of this writing, the issue is not resolved.

Insurance has become big business and really not even a business that must abide by the traditional trademarks of good business, i.e., honesty, flexibility, innovative thought, and above all, desire to please the client. After all, who is the client? Admittedly in this scenario with a physician partner who runs his own small business, the insurer has come perilously close to actually infuriating the real client as opposed to the patient who is merely employed by the corporate client. But most of the time, the insurer has little incentive to bend over backward for the individual patient.

The stories of wasted time and thwarted effort from any practitioner in this country are endless. Frustration no longer adequately describes the feelings of many. Some physicians would prefer a completely socialized system to this, where at least there would be only one payor—the government—to deal with, and that payor would at least be somewhat responsible to the voters. Insurance companies, by contrast, are responsible only to stockholders—and stockholders want profits.

# Noneconomic Damages

---

*Our litigation nightmare has extended to all industries and all walks of life. It is devouring our nation's productivity and making us less competitive in the world market. There's not much relief in sight because our legislatures are either full of attorneys, many of whom make a good living from personal injury litigation, or accept substantial campaign support from trial attorneys' organizations. The Clinton administration bill proposed in the fall of 1993 would have removed caps on mental anguish nationally that are now in place in some states. Since then, many different forms of national tort-reform legislation have been proposed. (As of 2006, the United States Congress has failed to pass a single piece of legislation restricting any fundamental aspect of civil litigation. In January of 2006, the request from the White House for tort-reform legislation was once again mentioned in the State of the Union address.)*

*While our litigation crisis increases malpractice premiums, drives the spread of costly defensive medicine practices, and undermines trust in physicians as a whole, it has a more insidious, destructive effect as it eats away at the joy of practicing medicine. Soon, there will be no reason to risk everything, every day, for anybody.*

---

Until near the end of my residency in 1985, I honestly thought *torts* were something that you ate, rather than vice versa. I now recognize that the food has an *e* on the end, and the legal term deals with a civil litigation in which the defendant physician may in fact be the only thing consumed. The litigation crisis may not be news to anyone, but the way in which it directly affects your health care might be.

We live in a society being destroyed by the erosion of individual responsibility. Consider the following:

- The wayward teen who rapes or murders or steals or sells drugs is now viewed as the unfortunate victim of societal circumstance. Somehow we have let them down, and so their behavior is less reprehensible.

- When a three-year-old gets run over by a truck at 11:00 p.m., it's no longer the parents who are responsible but clearly the maker of the insufficiently bright luminescent paint on the tricycle that failed to adequately protect the child.

- When a patient smokes cigarettes for forty years and gets lung cancer, it's not his responsibility despite the clear warning label stating that cigarette smoking may cause lung cancer, heart disease, birth defects, and even death. No, the manufacturer failed to warn him adequately that the nicotine in the cigarette might be habit-forming.

- When a woman gets breast cancer, it's not just bad luck, bad genes, and/or her failure to follow recommendations of breast self-exam and mammography that are responsible for the stage of disease at discovery. No, the last physician she saw is responsible for failing to diagnose her.

We have all heard the absurd stories of litigation brought by criminals falling through skylights or grossly obese people "emotionally injured" by a restaurant, airline, or theater that lacks seats into which they could comfortably fit. But these suits could not be brought in the absence of liberal juries and liberal judges who view large corporations as well-insured, deserving targets; magistrates who permit the filing of totally unfounded actions that defy common sense; and people willing to fill the role of plaintiff in order to get rich out of someone else's misfortune.

Medicine is only the very visible tip of the iceberg. The litigation crisis is undermining this country's productivity and siphoning its life blood into the coffers of large, flourishing law firms. Corporate funds are spent in increasing amounts to defend frivolous suits. The world's ten largest pharmaceutical companies have all moved overseas to avoid the huge legal costs of headquartering in the United States.

While corporations are affected by legal fees and costly product alterations undertaken to avoid litigation, medicine is affected both directly and indirectly as well. Obviously, rising costs of malpractice coverage were once passed on to consumers, but this represented only the most minor effect on medicine. In fact, that effect might be even less than ever because in 2006 as the malpractice premiums rise there is *no way* for your doctor to pass those costs on to you as the patient. (Ninety-eight percent of payments from third parties are negotiated discounts per procedure. In short, the insurer dictates compensation to a large extent. Rising malpractice insurance costs simply add more and more to the rising overhead of the average physician with no way to defray that cost.)

I believe there are three major mechanisms by which the litigation crisis directly influences the quality of your health care: first, costly defensive medicine practices; second, the creation of a quandary for the managed care physician who is losing decision-making authority; and third, the creation of a state of mind in your physician that is incompatible with optimum functioning.

The Clinton administration estimated $6 billion in defensive medicine costs for 1994. The American Medical Association estimated $100 billion. As of 2006, the estimate was more than twice that! My guess is that any estimate you pick is too low. Defensive medicine practices are so ingrained that they are not even consciously recognized as such. Much of the preoperative, admission, and antenatal testing done currently as routine could be completely eliminated from a purely medical standpoint. But in a society where perfect outcomes are not just expected but *demanded*—or else—these expenditures will continue. David Studdert, LLB, ScD, MPH, et al., in their excellent review, *Medical Malpractice*, list five central reasons for the sky-rocketing numbers of claims and size of awards: first, increased public awareness of medical errors; second, lower levels of confidence and trust in the health care system due to negative interaction with managed care; third, advances in innovative diagnostic technology; fourth, rising public expectations of perfect outcomes; and finally, greater reluctance among plaintiff attorneys to accept offers that in the past would have settled cases (*The New England Journal of Medicine*, Jan. 29, 2004, pp. 283–292).

If you walk into the emergency room tomorrow night and tell them you have the worst headache you've ever had in your life, you won't get out of there for less than $2,000. Now, the likelihood of your having a malignant brain tumor is extremely small. A full physical exam, including a blood pressure test, an eye exam, an ear exam, and a neurologic exam, would be adequate to assess and treat your headache. If you have no apparent neurologic signs, such as visual changes, slurred speech, or weakness in an extremity, then in the past you would have been discharged with some pain medication to see how things progressed over the next twelve to twenty-four hours.

Sounds simple, but that won't happen. Instead, unless you flat out refuse, you will get a CAT scan and/or MRI, and in all probability a lumbar puncture. Even if you refuse, you'll be asked to sign a form saying you left against medical advice. The ER doc just can't take the 6-in-100,000 chance that you're the one with the tumor (American Cancer Society, 2005–2006 statistics).

Let's take an example closer to home for a gynecologist. Other than hearing of a worrisome finding on her mammogram, there are probably no words a woman dreads more than, "Your Pap came back abnormal." Ever since George Papanicolaou designed the screening test for cervical cancer in the 1920s, an abnormal finding has been synonymous with possible precancerous disease of the cervix. Some of the mystery surrounding this particular killer has been resolved with the recognition of the causative role played by the sexually transmitted HPV. Those individuals who are virginal, celibate, or monogamous can now be reassured that they are at lower risk. But just as we achieve a better understanding, defensive medicine rears its ugly head in an unexpected way.

This is America. If a woman gets cervical cancer, she makes three calls: her husband, her mother, and her attorney. Plaintiff's attorneys have become increasingly savvy. They know that "abnormal" is a broad term that encompasses cells on a slide that may have nothing to do with precancerous changes, and that such cells can be found on almost half of all Paps. The vagina is full of bacteria. The uterus is sterile. Since the cervix connects the two, it is by definition full of inflammatory cells. These inflammatory cells can mimic very, very early precancerous cells.

So, if an unfortunate young woman gets invasive cervical cancer, an expert witness is paid to find any abnormal cell on a slide five years ago that was reported as normal, and the corporation that owns the pathology lab can just shell out $10–20 million regardless of the patient's treatment and prognosis.

Naturally, the nation's pathologists have moved to protect themselves from the rising tide of litigation. Instead of reading only 1–3% of Paps as abnormal with another 5% labeled "normal but with inflammatory atypia or reactive change," now they read 8% or so as abnormal but with a slightly different terminology applied. The 5% formerly labelled normal with inflammation are now reported as abnormal but with ASCUS or atypical squamous cells of undetermined significance. In short, the new Bethesda classification for Paps, in place since late 1992 and revised again in 2001, was developed to better communicate with practitioners but had the additional effect, intentional or not, of protecting pathologists from frivolous litigation. New liquid-based Pap smears screened initially by computer are definitely more sensitive than ever before. I'm all for that, except for one tiny little problem. There are human beings at the other end of these newly increased abnormal Pap rates. Guess who gets to call them with those frightening words?

The current recommendation from the American College of Obstetricians and Gynecologists is to re–Pap all non-precancerous abnormals in three to six months while at the same time performing more extensive testing with colposcopy (fancy binoculars) and biopsy if indicated.[1] Sounds logical, but it's cold comfort to the terrified patient who wants to know why she can't come back *tomorrow*, if not sooner, for a repeat (cells take months to turn over, inflammation can be treated, etc.). Colposcopy is expensive and time consuming as well. Furthermore, with the liability shifted so neatly to the gynecologist, many of them are simply choosing to grossly overtreat with expensive office lasers or electrical excision procedures rather than wait for the changes to resolve. Many labs in 2006 performed a reflex DNA probe to look for the presence of the most aggressive subtypes of HPV, yet physicians still sometimes opt to treat recurrent ASCUS even if HPV negative or in the absence of that information. (Over 70% of women who acquire the aggressive HPV subtypes in their cervix but who are under age thirty will clear the virus themselves within eighteen months without any treatment.) So once again, external forces come into play to warp the physician's judgment to the detriment of the patient. Defensive medicine costs are underestimated due to scenarios such as this. Their contribution to spiraling costs is not always as up-front as doing an MRI for a headache.

One more example: let's suppose that you have a pregnant patient who's scared of ultrasound or, even more likely, an insurance company that won't pay for it. In any event, the patient doesn't get an ultrasound exam at any point in pregnancy, and the baby is subsequently born with an ultrasound-identifiable defect, such as spina bifida or tetralogy of fallot (a common heart defect) or short-limbed dwarfism. If you haven't thoroughly documented the reason you didn't insist on an ultrasound exam and specifically mention the need to rule out this disease and haven't clearly documented the patient's refusal to have one performed, then you're in deep you-know-what.

While we're talking about documentation, here's a tiny example of how the litigation crisis is keeping us from caring for our patients appropriately. My daughter was born in 1988. Her mom's hospital chart was four pages. In 2006, at the same hospital, her hospital chart for a normal, uncomplicated vaginal delivery would be sixty-three pages! Form after form after form initially intended to clarify and document and avoid errors has now become a spider web of redundancy and opportunity for documentation error that actually opens the door to litigation rather than keeping it closed and steals valuable nursing and physician time from direct patient care.

Let's expand this point to include our second harmful effect of over-litigation, the quandary of the physician in managed care. Let's suppose the patient's managed-choice PPO does not pay for routine ultrasound. Furthermore, let's suppose that this Kroger grocery store checkout girl is not loaded with cash. When her baby has an obvious spina bifida that was sono-diagnosable, do you think the insurance company becomes the defendant? No way. The insurer can only be held liable for the original cost of the claim. After all, the insurer told her they wouldn't *pay* for a sonogram, not that she couldn't have one. It was the *physician* who should have told her how important it was to a safe outcome.

Physicians in a myriad of managed care scenarios are being forced to make suboptimal care decisions by insurers but are then held accountable for anything other than a perfect outcome. If they make the appropriate diagnostic decisions, it will either cost the patient out of her pocket or, as in many networks where patients are not allowed to pay for any services beyond the approved ones, it will have to be done at no charge. If the physician knuckles under and allows the insurer to dictate to him, there will be no sympathetic defense when a potentially diagnosable defect shows up. It is a no-win situation for patient and physician. (As mentioned in the foreword to this edition, some HMOs have now been held accountable for medical decisions, and lawsuits against the insurer along with the physician and hospital [of course] are on the rise.)

Finally, the current litigation crisis causes a huge number of formerly effective physicians to simply deteriorate due to their own mental anguish. While "mental anguish" is usually a term used to describe the nonfinancial damages suffered by a plaintiff from a wrongful action, it could equally be applied to the state of the defendant physician's thought processes.

Physicians are human, and their state of mind is reflected in their performance. For the most part, physicians also have a tremendous sense of responsibility, or they wouldn't spend eight to twelve years of their lives working for literally minimum wage for 120 hours a week in order to learn how to best help you.

Now, let's superimpose this sense of responsibility on the accusation that some specific act of omission or commission harmed a patient. Every physician is familiar with the Hippocratic credo, *primum non nocere*—first, do no harm. If in fact one lives his professional life by this medical golden rule, what do you suppose the psychological repercussions of such an accusation might be? I suppose it would be somewhat like telling Captain Picard or Captain Kirk that they purposefully flouted the prime directive and allowed the crew of the *Enterprise* to interfere with an advancing culture. Or better yet, if Captain Jack Sparrow refused to honor the pirate's code!

Never mind whether a mistake was actually made or not, and, of course, in medicine, that question is often open to interpretation. What would be the repercussions of such an accusation on an honest, dedicated physician? I can tell you. I've been there. Imagine how you would feel if you received a card in the mail from an angry parent who tells you she can't tolerate the thought that *your* children are healthy, but because of your incompetence, hers is not.

Mental anguish is the answer. It comes in all forms, and it camps at your mental doorstop for a very long time indeed. First there is the self-doubt, the self-questioning. Could I have done better? Did I really make the error I am accused of, and if so, did it really lead to the outcome? Did I do something, even inadvertently, that hurt or injured or killed my patient?

Doctors ask themselves these questions all the time. They're asked in the shower, they're asked on the highway, they're asked while tossing and turning and trying to sleep, they're asked when your kids are trying to get your attention, they're asked while ignoring your spouse's need for comfort or support, they're asked while seeing an office patient who brings the topic to mind, or they're asked while you're operating or sitting in church or singing in the choir or while you're supposed to be teaching Sunday school.

They're asked when you're supposed to be relaxing out to dinner or a movie or a cocktail party. They're asked while you throw a ball to your dog or mow the lawn or while you're apologizing to your wife for the hundredth time because you didn't hear what she said. These questions go round and round and round in your head sometimes for months at a time. They preoccupy you while you wait for the possible suit after a tragic outcome. They hang over you after notification of a suit to be filed in ninety days. They vex you before, during, and after depositions. They hunt you down before and after trial or settlement.

And don't let me kid you, these aren't the only questions. Because even if you're eventually convinced that your action or inaction did not lead to the poor outcome, there are questions in your mind about your *own* outcome.

What will this do to the most important thing I have, my reputation?

# Noneconomic Damages

What if I lose everything I've saved for my kids and my wife? What if the case comes to trial and we get a jury so empathetic with the plight of the plaintiff that the medical facts are ignored and they find a judgment against me for more than my insurance limits? Do I declare bankruptcy? I wonder what's involved with that? Can they attach my wages forever so that *I'll never get through this?*

There are new dangers as well. As the National Practitioner Data Bank, which records malpractice suit information, is made public, physicians may be de-selected from HMO and PPO provider panels on the basis of one settlement. Already proposed National Committee for Quality Assurance data would eliminate providers with one case settled for $30,000 dollars or more in the last five years. This will preselect providers who are younger and less experienced. Further, it will penalize the patients of thousands of excellent physicians who settled cases out of court rather than endure the torture of years of litigation even if the issue was one of legitimate clinical judgment.

In many states, including Texas, a single anonymous complaint to the Board of Medical Examiners can launch an investigation whereby *one* instance determined to represent substandard care (i.e., one error in clinical judgment established retrospectively from an adverse outcome) can encumber your license to practice medicine. In a managed care environment, even a former slap on the wrist, such as mandatory continuing medical education (CME) for a brief period, can cause a physician to be removed from HMO provider panels. If, say, 70% of his patients are managed care, that slap on the wrist amounts to the same thing as revocation of his license!

Imagine going to work every day in a situation where there is *zero* tolerance for error. In short, despite being human, you are simply not permitted to make a mistake, or it may cost you everything you have in the world.

It's of course ridiculous. But that's what the American physician lives with every day. In an instant-gratification society, a society that sees miraculous, new, high technology every day, the concept of a bad outcome has become unacceptable. If things just don't turn out the way they're expected to, somebody's responsible and somebody must pay.

Well, somebody is paying, and it's not just the physician, it's the patient as well.

You're paying because your doctor is forced to do things that are medically unnecessary, so that he can try to protect himself.

You're paying because your doctor is being forced into a situation where someone else really makes the medical decisions under the guise of deciding what will be covered, and yet he retains most, if not all, of the liability.

You're paying because your doctor is dealing with emotions and stresses that shouldn't be there, and those emotions can affect his judgment and performance in a very real way.

So what can be done?

There are some simple answers. The rest of the civilized world from Japan to Germany has figured it out. First, make the plaintiff pay all costs if he or she loses. This will seriously limit frivolous suits.

Second, don't allow contingency fees. Force lawyers to work like everyone else—for a fee. In legitimate cases, the damages then go where they belong—to the plaintiff.

Third, limit awards for pain and suffering. If no price can be set on intangibles, don't let juries or judges put absurdly high ones in place. As of 2006, many states, including Texas, have finally put limitations on mental anguish, also known as noneconomic damages. Still these limits are usually between a quarter of a million dollars and a million dollars for *each* defendant. If a suit involves two physicians, a nurse and a hospital for instance, bingo, you're up to a million dollars for pain and suffering right out of the chute!

Fourth, allow juries to know about alternate compensation. In many states, the plaintiff standing before the jury may already be a millionaire due to compensation from other defendants' settlements or insurance payouts. When a jury is instructed to extrapolate lost wages for the estimated working lifetime of the plaintiff, it is superfluous if the injured party has already been compensated from another codefendant for the same thing. In other words, lost income should only be calculated once, then split among the defendants, not paid out over and over by each defendant.

The litigation crisis took a backseat to the shifting paradigm in which the physician's decision-making power was being eroded in the 1990s, but it's back on the front burner again in 2006. In the late 1980s and through much of the 1990s physicians and hospitals could generally pass on malpractice premium hikes directly to the consumer. But now, with the spread of managed–care contracting, tight cost controls on Medicare, and the adoption of restrictive fee schedules by private insurers, net incomes are dropping precipitously for physicians. While I don't expect you to shed many tears over that, realize that malpractice premiums have so eaten into many Ob/Gyns' incomes that over 10% per year are quitting obstetrics and many are seeking early retirement or alternate careers. And there are new dangers as well. The new breed of health care provider may be employed by a big HMO corporation. His malpractice premiums may be paid as part of his compensation. As he adopts the casual attitude of the shift worker, coming to work at nine and leaving at five, seeing rotating patients every day, he may not go that little extra mile to ensure the best outcome. After all, he's only one of many physicians that may care for a particular patient. It's not like he's solely responsible for your health anyway!

Besides, who ya' gonna sue? The corporation, where the deep pockets are. I just work here, lady.*

---

* Most HMOs did not permit themselves to be sued for malpractice. All patients, as part of their contracts, had to sign and agree to binding arbitration, even if unknowingly. The courts began to change this in the late 1990s, and HMOs became targets of plaintiff attorneys as well.

# Something Bad Wrong

---

*Managed care, whether "managed" by an insurance industry intent on profit or by the federal government intent on a misguided, misconceived notion of guaranteed comprehensive health care for everyone, is fraught with danger. There ain't no free lunch.*

*Our legislators' self-imposed moral imperative—to provide health care for everyone—has run up against simple economics: somebody has to pay. In order for the insurance companies or the government to guarantee that their proposed paradigms will function, they must obtain control of as many variables as possible. They must control both providers and patients, and in the government's case, misguided egalitarianism may lead to equally rationed mediocre care for all of us.*

*Such plans would entail tremendous cost financially (the 1993 "Clinton plan" would have cost $1 trillion in new spending over the next eight years, according to the Congressional Budget Office) and tremendous cost in quality with millions of people forced into plans they don't want that restrict their choices and undermine their doctor's ability to make decisions.*

*With the failure of the Clinton health care reform effort in the fall of 1994, the future of reform is anything but clear. The Health-insurance Portability and Accountability Act of 1996 (HIPAA) along with Medicare cuts as part of the Balanced Budget Act of 1997, and most recently Medicare Part D (prescription drug coverage), are as close as*

# Something Bad Wrong

*Congress has gotten to even approaching the topic by 2006. Arguably, and we will discuss it later, these attempts may have made things worse and not better anyway.*

*But I want to show you how changes already wrought by managed care in the 1990s are affecting you daily. Institutionalizing these changes by law will simply hasten the destruction of the entire system, a destruction already well on its way.*

---

K atie, you know where my patient is by any chance?" I continued to randomly flip over, turn around, and otherwise mess up charts in the rack and on the nurse's desk.

"Twy in twelve, Docta. You wememba, the pelvic woom?" The no-nonsense head nurse of the graveyard shift in the emergency room swept around the corner with a pen clenched in her teeth, an IV and angiocath in one hand and a liter of saline in the other.

"Oh, you mean just like always for the last twenty-one years?" I asked innocently as Katie rocketed down the hallway towards a trauma room.

She glanced back over her shoulder and hollered, somewhat impeded by her oral grasp of the Bic, "How do you ewer fine your own socks, Docta?"

I picked the metal clipboard out of the plexiglass slot marked "12" and glanced over it as I walked quickly down the gray linoleum hall. Without looking up, I negotiated the gurneys and wheelchairs much as a trained marine would a familiar obstacle course. The various conveyances held the usual assortment of disoriented elderly, inebriated, and lacerated street people, screaming children with everything from ear infections to broken limbs as well as anxious, overweight people in their sixties with oxygen masks in place, worrying about heart attacks.

# Disrobe Completely

At the end of the hall, I turned right to a cul-de-sac with three exam rooms. All were designated as female rooms, purportedly because they contained the necessary equipment considered the stock and trade of my specialty. Tonight, the door to 11 stood open. A youngish redhead with an IV in her arm sat on the end of the bed, vomiting into a trash can held by an unhappy male who had his head turned to the side. The sound of her heaving was overwhelming and unstoppable, like a diesel truck shifting gears on a steep grade. I said a brief silent prayer of thanks that this was not my patient, since I am one of those empathetic vomiters who simply cannot be in the same room with an upchucker.

I pushed open the door to 12 and immediately saw that Suzanne Rogers was not in a good way. She had called earlier in the day, complaining of severe abdominal pain. A nurse had told her that since she was on the pill, her last period was on time, and her pain was on her left side, that it probably wasn't anything serious—maybe a muscle strain or something. But the pain kept getting worse, so I had asked them to meet me at the hospital.

Now Suzanne lay on her right side, knees curled up and moaning. Her hospital gown was soaked with sweat. Her dishwater-blond hair lay limply across her face. Her eyes, half open, focused only after I spoke. "Fancy meeting you here at 1:30 in the morning! Couldn't sleep either? We could've just done lunch you know!" My quip brought only the weakest of smiles to her face.

"Hi, Doctor T! Am I glad to see you! Nobody around here seems to take me seriously." Each word was pseudowhispered as if the breath required for normal volume was too painful to contemplate. Her husband sat nervously fidgeting on the edge of a plastic chair at the foot of the bed, his arm outstretched to rub her foot.

"There's something bad wrong with her, doc," he said. "These folks here say it's just a ruptured cyst, but I don't know. She don't look right to me. Never been a time she didn't read a story to one of the kids at bedtime, and I did 'em both tonight while she soaked in the tub. It just got worse after that. Then she started throwin' up and moanin' and carryin' on, and I got scared."

Suzanne had been my patient for at least seven years. I delivered both their six-year-old daughter and their four-year-old son. She was not a powder puff. Both of her deliveries had been unmedicated, and her performance had been as perfect as Katerina Witt skating to her second gold medal. Her husband was right. For her to look like this, something bad was going on.

Gently, I helped her roll onto her back. I listened to the total silence in all four quadrants of her belly where bowel sounds should have been. Just tapping on her lower tummy, especially the left, brought a wince and a yelp of agony. There was no doubt; something was causing a peritonitis. A ruptured appendix? Less likely with pain starting on the left and then spreading, but still never lower than third on the list of possibilities. Could have been a ruptured cyst, as the intern had suggested to them, but you don't often get cysts on the birth control pill, and, besides, Suzanne just looked too sick.

I took her pulse at the wrist. 122! Pretty far up there to be sustained by pain alone. The sweating and the pallor all fit with the onset of shock secondary to intra-abdominal bleeding. In the absence of a ruptured spleen caused by a direct blow, ectopic pregnancy had to be number one on the list. I asked her a few more questions about her history and got all the information I needed from her and her husband.

"You're gonna be alright, kiddo," I told her. "We'll get you something for pain, I'll check some lab results, and I'll be right back." I stroked my hand over her sweat-soaked brow and gave her husband a wink for reassurance.

Once outside, I called the OR and told them to get ready for possible laparoscopy, but more likely an emergency laparotomy for a ruptured ectopic pregnancy. They said they'd alert anesthesia for me. I collared the intern whose name was on the chart as he came out of the X-ray reading room behind the desk. After brief introductions, I told him I had some quick questions about the lady in room 12.

"Oh, the ruptured cyst?"

"You got the adjective correct, but I believe the noun incorrect."

His look was somewhere between incredulity and annoyance. "Look, it's 2:00 a.m. Just spell it out."

"You took that lady's history, didn't you?" He admitted that he had, in addition to doing a very painful pelvic exam.

"What's the first thing you always ask any male ER patient over the age of eighteen?" The intern had no problem with that one. He responded as we all could from rote, "Are you now, or have you ever been, in the service of any branch of the Armed Forces of the United States?" Even if the man was in a drunken stupor, an affirmative answer would get him an ambulance ride to the nearest VA Hospital.

"Now, what's the first thing you ask any girl or woman over the age of twelve who presents with abdominal pain?"

He knew that one, too. "When was your last period? But I asked her that. It was right on time and a pill withdrawal at that. She's had no irregular bleeding not even spotting, and she's never missed a pill by her story." The intern seemed a little smug at his success so far.

"What kind of pill is she on?"

"I didn't ask. So what?"

"What other meds is she on?"

"I guess I didn't ask." A little less smug now.

"Well, I'll tell you. . . . Katie, call the lab and add a serum pregnancy test to 12's lab, *stat*, will ya? And keep a nurse in there all the time for the next few minutes. Oh, and open up her IV and type and cross her for four units. . . . Now, where were we?"

"Other meds."

"Oh, yes. She was supposed to be on a 1/50 pill because of her anticonvulsant meds and their interference with estrogen metabolism."

"Oops. I guess she wasn't, huh?" The intern looked a little like a puppy who's just spotted the rolled-up newspaper in your hand.

"Here's the part you're gonna love. Her HMO refused to pay for that brand of pills. They only have three brands on their formulary, so they substituted a generic 1/20 when she got her three-month supply of pills in the mail. She questioned the color change on the phone to the pharmacy, but they assured her the insurer would only have substituted a generic equivalent. Incidentally, it's illegal to do that in this state unless I specifically allow substitution, which I wouldn't have in her case. I'll bet you dollars to donuts she's bleeding like a stuck pig inside from a ruptured left ectopic pregnancy."

"Well, let me know what you find, and, ah, thanks." The intern shuffled to the rack and grabbed the next chart. It seemed like only yesterday that I lived in his twilight world of near-total sleeplessness.

Needless to say, Suzanne had to have her left tube removed. If we'd caught it earlier, we might have saved it, but without knowing she was pregnant, Suzanne hadn't been in for any early testing.

There are three separate ways in which managed care could have killed Suzanne Rogers.

First, the obviously inappropriate and illegal substitution of a non-equivalent prescription drug in the interests of cost cutting.

Second, had Suzanne been forced to see a physician unfamiliar with her history of pain tolerance with natural childbirth, the doctor might not have held a high enough index of suspicion of an intra-abdominal catastrophe. He might also have missed her history of anticonvulsant use and not thought to actually check on the identity of her oral contraceptive.

Third, even had Suzanne suspected a pregnancy, under a managed care plan she would have had to waste time seeing her designated internist primary-care provider before being allowed to see her Ob/Gyn. As it was, her insurance company—unbelievably—*denied payment* for her ruptured ectopic, retroactively claiming that she in fact bypassed her primary-care provider in not seeing him earlier in her pregnancy. The fact that she was unaware of her pregnancy did not sway them nor that the operation was lifesaving and emergent. The outpatient surgery cost them well over $10,000, less than a third of which was physicians' fees. As far as I know, the patient and her husband, a dairy farmer, are still fighting the good fight with her insurer. We actually charged her only 50% of our usual fee and adjusted the rest off. The hospital was evidently feeling less generous, and if her insurer chose not to come through, they would have to come up with the full amount eventually.

Such stories abound. Recently, a patient of mine was driven to my office at 4:00 p.m. on a Friday. She was bleeding heavily and cramping severely and believed she was in the midst of a miscarriage. After looking at her card, my receptionist informed her that she should be aware her insurer required her to see her primary-care provider first, or they would deny pregnancy-related claims.

The patient, despite her misery, called the 800-number from the lobby. She got an operator in Connecticut who told her there were no available appointments for ten days with her acceptable providers. After she patiently explained the emergent nature of the problem, they looked up an alternative MD on the computer and told her a network doctor in Winnsboro (one hundred miles east of Dallas) could see her in half an hour. She told them unless they wanted to pay for a LifeFlight helicopter, it seemed unlikely that she'd be able to get there.

But (insane) rules are rules. It was the only option they would provide. I saw the patient in the office for nothing. She required a D&C, which the hospital allowed her to pay off over time.

Many managed care plans now require women to get an authorization from their primary-care provider (PCP) in the form of a referral number before they can see their Ob/Gyn. A twenty-nine-year-old patient of mine called her

# Something Bad Wrong

Managed Choice PCP, which just happened to be a woman internist located forty-six miles from where she lives and works. She asked for a referral number to be allowed to see me, her Ob/Gyn of six years, for new onset mid-cycle bleeding and pain with intercourse. She was denied by the internist's office, being informed that she had already received one authorization only two months previously. The fact that the previous referral was to an ophthalmologist for an eye infection, they claimed, had no relevance. My patient reluctantly acquiesced and made the trek to see the internist.

When the patient called me, hysterical and in tears later that afternoon, she related an unfortunately all-too-common scenario. The internist had painfully inserted the speculum and examined her vagina for six minutes. When apparently unable to visualize the cervix, she asked my patient if she'd had a hysterectomy! My patient, somewhat taken aback, replied that she had not. Was something wrong? The internist proceeded with a bimanual pelvic exam and told her that she also couldn't feel her ovaries. The errors were compounded by subsequent statements about my patient's potential for infertility problems due to her abnormal anatomy, questions about her husband's fidelity in light of her pain and bleeding, cultures for sexually transmitted diseases, and blood tests for suspected hormonal abnormalities.

All of this was bologna. The bleeding was caused by a problem rectified by changing her pill. The pain was caused by the most common type of vaginal infection other than yeast, easily treated with a cream. Her anatomy was totally normal, as later documented in my office with vaginal sonography at no cost to put her mind at ease.

For women under fifty, 90% of health care needs involve the reproductive organs, breasts, or reproductive hormones. Internists get six *weeks* of training in this area and while your Ob/Gyn has four to six *years*. Should women be denied access to their Ob/Gyns in a misguided, unproven attempt at cost containment? What about gynecological procedures like colposcopy to follow up abnormal Paps, electrosurgical and laser cone biopsies of the cervix, hysteroscopy to see into the uterus, endometrial biopsies, Depo-Provera birth control injections, Norplant placement and removal, IUD placement and removal, and even birth-control pill management with over sixty pills on the market with eleven different progestins in all different ratios to multiple different doses of estrogen? Internists and family practitioners in different parts of the country have assumed all of these responsibilities with little or no training under the auspices of restrictive HMOs mandating gatekeeper systems that do not designate the Ob/Gyn as the provider of women's health care.

In 1994, 30% of all HMOs did not allow a woman self-referral to her own gynecologist.[2] Furthermore, capitated systems, which we'll examine more closely shortly, financially penalize the family practitioner or internist for referring to the specialist, Ob/Gyn or otherwise. HMOs may argue this as cost-effective and preventive medicine, but much data suggests otherwise.

According to the National Ambulatory Medical Care Survey in 1990, annual exams by gynecologists were twice as likely to include a Pap smear, three times as likely to include a pelvic exam, and twice as likely to include a breast exam. Competence aside, if the internist or family practitioner is either too busy or too uncomfortable to even perform a complete physical, including the parts of the woman's body most likely to harbor dangerous disorders, is it good preventive medicine even if someone can show a cost savings?

And could you be expected to show a true savings in the long run when accounting for delayed diagnosis and consequent increased expense for breast, cervical, uterine, and ovarian cancers? What about early diagnosis of ectopic pregnancy before rupture, endometriosis, or ovarian tumors?

I have a question for you husbands out there who advocate a restrictive HMO because it saves you a couple hundred dollars in the next year even though it doesn't permit your wife to see her gynecologist. Would you let her get on an airliner flown by a pilot who you knew had only six weeks of experience flying Piper Cubs before he stepped into the cockpit of the 767?

The United States House of Representatives passed a 1994 resolution "expressing the sense of the House . . . that Ob/Gyns should be designated as primary-care providers for women in federal laws relating to the provision of health care." Delaware, Georgia, and Virginia have passed similar resolutions. California passed a law in September 1994 requiring payers to consider Ob/Gyns primary-care providers. Maryland and New York have passed laws that require payers to allow women direct access to their Ob/Gyns for at least one visit per year.[3] But still most states have no such protections for women's access to their Ob/Gyns. (While the numbers are better in 2006, still many states have no such provisions.)

Many managed care plans now require their patients to get referrals from their PCP for each OB visit during their pregnancy. Furthermore, my office staff needs an average of four different precertification codes for just a vaginal delivery, all requiring separate phone exchanges throughout the pregnancy. Failure to follow the rules of each insurer, which literally change daily, can result in nonpayment.

But the dangers are not in any way limited to restrictions on availability. Cost containment by an outside agency that does not have the patient's welfare as its primary concern can have a direct negative effect on outcome.

Case in point: just this week one of my patients delivered twins at twenty-nine weeks—three months early. During the previous three weeks, I had carried on no less than five phone conversations with her insurer. In the final call two weeks ago, I was again denied approval for home monitoring on the basis that the patient had not already been hospitalized and treated for preterm labor.

The whole point in the management of twins, of course, is prevention. Multiple gestation starts out as high risk for preterm delivery by definition.

# Disrobe Completely

Once preterm labor begins, it may be impossible to stop, but home monitoring of uterine contractions with telephone transmission of the tracings may identify the process early enough for treatment to be effective. Even much cheaper daily phone contact with a nurse might head off preterm delivery.

The cost to the insurer would have been $150 per day for the monitor or even less for daily nursing contact. That may seem like a lot until you consider the *$3,500 a day* they will pay for at least the next fifty to sixty days of neonatal intensive care unit (NICU). You may note that comes to around $210,000! Well, here is reform at work. This is certainly "value enhancement." (Interestingly, in 1998, home uterine monitoring was shown to be ineffective; this was not, however, the case in 1995, and ineffectiveness was not the purported reason for denial of payment.)

If my patient had been able to follow my recommendation without the interference of her insurance bureaucracy, she not only might have saved the system huge expense, but also might have had her twins go home with her instead of spend weeks on ventilators. With the excellent (but costly) care they will receive from the neonatal intensive care unit (NICU), they stand a good chance of not developing the chronic pulmonary, renal, intestinal, and hearing problems frequently associated with the premature, but only time will tell.

Two years ago, a forty-eight-year-old patient of mine was in for a yearly exam. Since her mother, sister, and an aunt had all died of ovarian cancer, I consented to allow her a blood test called a CA-125. The test is designed to follow response to therapy with known cancers that produce this marker. Admittedly, it is not indicated as a screening test for ovarian cancer. Even though the test is only 60–80% sensitive at detecting cancer, any help in early diagnosis might be worthwhile, given her strong family history. Only later did I discover that when she was told at the front desk that the $125 test would not be covered by her HMO, she elected to forego it.

You know where this is going. Fourteen months later when she returned slightly late for her annual exam, I found a mass in her left ovary. This was confirmed by office ultrasound, and subsequently her CA-125 was found to be extremely high. Her disease had spread throughout her abdominal cavity, dooming her to both the discomforts of chemo and radiotherapy and the certain prognosis of death on the very near horizon.

Now, no one can say that her disease was confined to one ovary (curable by removal of the ovary). Fourteen months before or even that, her CA-125 would have been positive. But if both of these things were true, her care would have been much cheaper, and oh, yes, she'd still be alive.

On any given day, I can now ask any physician colleague who is in active practice to recount the managed care nightmare he experienced that same day! Today, for instance, I passed through the lounge on the way from a surgery to the locker room and heard two doctor acquaintances exchanging stories from earlier in the same day. One had been denied approval on a blood test to determine whether a woman was carrying the gene for Duchenne muscular dystrophy (DMD).

The patient's brother had DMD, and her sister was a carrier of the X-linked recessive disorder. She was aware of a 50% chance that she carried the gene on one of her X chromosomes. If she was a carrier, then because any son of hers would get one of her X chromosomes, he would have a 50% chance of having the disease. And any daughter would have a 50% risk of being a carrier. However, if she did not carry the gene, her progeny's risk was zero.

Without carrier testing, the couple faced the 50% possibility of their child either carrying the gene or in fact having the disease with this discoverable only at amniocentesis. Then they would be faced with the choice of terminating their pregnancy or risking a life-shortening, debilitating disease in a son or potentially passing on the disease through a daughter. Therefore, carrier-testing to determine her status was appropriate.

To her doctor, that is. The medical director of the insurance company on final appeal stated that the test was not medically necessary. The medical director went on to say that as far as he was concerned, "reproduction itself is not medically necessary." (An interesting viewpoint, and I suppose defensible on an individual basis, but hard to accept from a species perspective!)

The other physician had just been denied the use of heparin, the only blood-thinner shown to be safe in pregnancy, for a woman who had nearly died with a massive pulmonary embolus in her last pregnancy. The insurance reviewer refused to pay for the medicine because it was not on their OB formulary. She suggested instead a drug that is strictly contraindicated and shown to cause severe birth defects in humans. Once this was pointed out, she simply responded that the medicine was not covered, and the "client" could foot the $1,500 bill herself if she wouldn't use their formulary choice.

Danger. There is demonstrable danger in removing health care decisions from the hands of patients and their physicians. Decisions about diagnosis and treatment should be dictated by the patient's needs and *not* by fiscal considerations. These decisions should not be dictated by forcing patients to go to gatekeepers or designated primary-care providers; by forced referral patterns or lack thereof with respect to specialists; by misguided, ill-informed, purse-string management of pharmaceuticals; or by restricting diagnostic laboratory and imaging tests thought necessary by the attending physician.

Ill-informed, purse-string management is not confined to the private sector. Recently, the National Cancer Institute (NCI) changed their recommendations for screening mammograms to start only at age fifty, overruling their own National Cancer Advisory Board![4] They did so purportedly on the basis of one roundly criticized Canadian study that concluded that survival time was not increased in woman under age fifty.[5,6,7,8,9,10] No other group bought into the study—not the American Cancer Society, not the American College of Surgeons, not the American College of Obstetricians and Genealogists, not the American College of Radiology. What a coincidence that only the federally funded NCI came up with a recommendation that would save the government hundreds of millions in Medicaid expenditures!

The Colorado Mammogram Advocacy Program (CMAP) has recorded the findings of every single mammogram performed in the state for a number of years. Guess what? More cancers were diagnosed in the forty-to-fifty age group than the fifty-to-sixty age group. In fact, about 30% of all the breast cancers detected were in woman under fifty.[11] Our own data at Presbyterian Hospital in Dallas corroborates this. Out of 27,249 mammograms performed since 1992, 234 patients were diagnosed with cancer. There were seventy breast cancers in women under fifty, or about 30%!

Follow the NCI's recommendation, and a huge number of these woman would have been diagnosed at a later stage and grade and consequently worsened prognosis.[12] All of the major medical societies have stuck with a recommendation of a first mammogram at thirty-five to forty, at least every other year from forty to fifty, and yearly from fifty on. But many insurance companies seem to like the National Cancer Institute's recommendations. All of a sudden, some insurers aren't covering mammogram for women in their forties. Who would society benefit more from saving: the forty-two-year-old working mother of small children or the seventy-five-year-old grandmother in questionable health?[13] (Incidentally, NCI has since changed their recommendation to be in line with the ACS and ACOG, i.e., yearly mammograms from age forty on.)

Danger. Let a respected institution like NCI be directed solely by cost concerns and not by health concerns, and people are going to die needlessly. For twenty years we've worked to make women aware of the importance of mammography, and in one ill-considered move, the NCI did irreparable damage to women and possibly fatal damage to some particular women.

But the danger inherent in these scenarios is nothing compared to that looming on the horizon in many parts of the country and in fact is already the case in other parts. By that, I mean the danger of the institutionally employed physician, wherein the institution is the contracting entity with employers and insurers.

Traditionally, or at least since World War II, insurers have contracted with individuals to cover some percentage of their health care costs after a deductible is met. As costs have risen, this paradigm has shifted such that employers contract with insurers, and the employee-patient is then directed to a PPO plan (preferred provider) with little or no deductible and a tiny co-pay, such as five to ten dollars.

The preferred providers aren't "preferred" in the traditional sense, of course; they're not chosen because they are known to practice good medicine necessarily, but only because they've signed a contract to accept reduced fees in exchange for the listing. Both hospitals and doctors play this game. All of the dangers enumerated above can rear their heads in this situation, but at least the physician is still autonomous, even if the patients' choices of doctors, drugs and hospitals are channeled.

But things can get worse. Enter "capitation." An ugly word for an ugly idea. Capitation is simply a per-capita system. An insurer will pay a contracting entity—let's say, for sake of argument, a hospital—a set amount per patient per month to cover all eventualities. Any money left over at the end of the fiscal year is profit for the hospital. If the hospital either employs or, by nature of the capitation contracts, substantially controls the physicians on its staff, their compensation too is tied to funds left over at the end of the year. The physician's individual productivity in dollars is tracked by computer and broken down into "fixed overhead" such as rent, utilities, insurance, etc., and "variable overhead" such as supplies, laboratory tests, imaging tests, consults with specialists, and hospitalizations.

It's easy to see what happens here. A system comes into being where both doctors and hospitals are rewarded for delivering *less* health care. Not better, not necessarily more efficient, but *less* health care. A financial incentive—which for the patient might, in fact, be a life and death financial incentive—is created to lower costs at all costs.

○○○

Several years ago I had lunch with the medical director of a nearby family practice group. They had formed their own HMO without walls and took almost 90% of their patients on capitation. During the usual tuna salad and iced tea fare in the hospital's conference room, I asked this sixty-year-old physician how his group handled referrals.

"What do you mean, referrals?"

"I mean, if a patient presents with a difficult arrhythmia and you want them to see a cardiologist, do you sub-contract that out or what?"

"We don't do that," he said with finality.

"You don't do what?" I said, thoroughly confused.

"We don't refer. To anyone. Ever."

"You mean you handle renal failure without a nephrologist, and seizure disorders without a neurologist, and ruptured discs without a surgeon?" I was incredulous.

"Exactly."

"Is that a good idea? I mean, are your patients really getting the best care?"

"Who said anything about the best care? That's not the game anymore, doctor. The bottom line is the game. There are twelve family practitioners in the group. We'd love to have your guys be our obstetrics arm. Currently that's the ONLY thing we sub out."

"But what if you just don't have the expertise to handle someone's problem? What if it's life threatening?"

He looked at me with what I can only describe as contempt. Wiping the mayonnaise off his chin and throwing his napkin on the plate, he abruptly pushed back his chair and stood up.

"I guess they should have thought about that when they bought cheap insurance!"

You'll be happy to know that we didn't join their merry little band. When I related this story to my brother, the heart surgeon, he laughed bitterly.

"My partner had a bitch of a month in June," he said. "Three out of six of his coronary bypass patients died either in or right after surgery. He was devastated. But not everybody was unhappy. The first week in July he got a certificate in the mail for being the 'low-cost provider' in cardiovascular surgery for the month of June!

"It's the God's honest truth!" he went on. "Even got a write-up in the HMO paper. 'Course no one mentioned that ICU time is *very* expensive, and if your patients die on the table it's extremely cost effective!"

This is danger with a capital D. At least in a one-party payor, socialized system, there's no *disincentive* for care. Sure, the government might totally screw things up and end up rationing health care in a big way; but at least under such a system the hospitals and doctors *theoretically* wouldn't be paid to under-diagnose and under-treat you. As we shall discuss shortly, however, there may be plenty of opportunities for a nationalized system to make sweeping decisions in the interest of cost containment that adversely affect the health of millions at a single blow!

It is true that various forms of managed care have successfully reduced health care costs for many large companies. But the outcome data for these changes in terms of patient satisfaction and overall quality of care is embryonic.

By 2006 outcome data is still a complicated, contentious mess, but one thing is clear, managed care is no longer cost effective for corporate America! In fact the burden of carrying health care benefits for the aging baby boomers at work and in pension funds is forcing former giants of industry to their knees, as we shall see!

# Teaching?

*There is another danger not to be underestimated. All medical schools depend on their urban medical center institutions as training grounds for medical students, interns and residents. These academic centers associated with medical schools are also the central nervous system for the country's medical research. Our institutions of higher learning in medical education are being seriously threatened by managed care.*

Teaching hospitals must now compete with non-academic institutions for the exploding number of managed care contract patients. They are being forced to negotiate rock-bottom prices for services, often below cost. As managed care sweeps the nation, both HMOs and hospitals are acquiring outpatient care facilities, physicians' practices, nursing homes, laboratories, etc., in an effort to ensure they are not left out of the market. As Dr. Jerome Kassirer points out, academic medical centers and managed care plans have very different missions.

"Managed-care organizations, particularly those owned by investors, are required only to apply existing knowledge to routine patient care. Academic medical centers, on the other hand, create new knowledge, develop and assess new technologies, evaluate new drugs, educate medical students, train tomorrow's physicians, and care for the sickest patients."[14]

Dr. Kassirer goes on to show that the costs of these programs combined with demographics of patient populations make the costs for these academic institutions 30–40% higher than the cost for competing proprietary or community hospitals. Managed-care organizations, with an eye solely to cost, avoid academic institutions for their patients. As a result, many such hospitals are being left over-bedded, underused, and in real danger of extinction.

If we undermine our nation's capacity to do basic research while at the same time diminishing our capacity to educate physicians, we will poison our own future. There is genuine reason to be alarmed at what profit-driven, managed care organizations may do to our academic institutions, albeit indirectly, and thus what they may do to our children's and grandchildren's health care.

We should continue to look for solutions to cost-containment issues that do not dismantle our current medical infrastructure and perhaps put obstacles in the way of what trained physicians know to be the optimum medical choices. At the same time, we must strive to avoid destroying our world-class academic institutions in the rush to hold down costs. The danger signs are proliferating, and it is time to take action.

"Let us not look back in anger, or forward in fear, but around us in awareness."

—James Thurber

# Part 4

# Scoot All the Way to the Edge:

## Approaches

*Don't get excited now. Don't go kiddin' yourself. The health care crisis is not going to dissipate under the influence of my startling intellect over the next several paragraphs. However, I would like to make what I feel to be a few valid observations, and then point us in a direction that stands the best chance of attaining health care reform without eliminating the best aspects of our current system.*

*What do we want? That's pretty easy. We want to keep our relationship with our doctors and let our doctors keep making the decisions about our care. But we want to halt the upward spiral of costs associated with the delivery of our health care while maintaining quality and, at the same time, improving access to the system for all income levels. Simple, right?*

*Before we can fix anything, a rudimentary understanding of what went wrong seems important. I believe there are five basic forces which combined to leave us in this mess, and we shall examine each one briefly.*

# The Problem

## Overview

America spends 13% of its gross domestic product (GDP) on health care, by far the highest in the world. The United States also spends the largest amount per capita on health care of any nation in the world ($4,178 in the United States versus $1,783 on average for industrialized nations in 1998, and $5,267 in the United States in 2002), yet we have over 45 million people who have no realistic, effective access to the system. With over 15% of our population uninsured, millions of people seek health care only when it becomes critical, and problems which could have been averted earlier and more cheaply are now terribly expensive.[14a]

Health-care costs are rising at the annual rate of roughly 14%. Employers nationwide report that they can only absorb about a 9% annual increase unless something gives. It was estimated in 2004 that on average, employers' costs for health care would increase by 54% over the next five years, forcing employee contributions to at least triple! (There's the "give.") Intense competition and overcapacity in many industries has made it impossible for them to pass the rising cost of health care on to customers. They are forced to pass it on to employees instead.

It has been estimated that between 19.1 and 24.3% of our total costs are administrative, due to our phenomenally cumbersome and complicated multiparty payor system.[14b]

Finally, the United States population is aging rapidly as the baby boomers reach retirement age, and the burdens on the system are sky-rocketing.

# The Problem

Given all that, many ask the question, "Does the U.S. even have the best health care system in the world?" as has so often been touted by myself and many others? With growing costs and less access for millions, on what basis can we claim to have the best system? The World Health Organization (WHO) released a revealing study in 2000 in which it analyzed and compared the health care delivery systems of its 191 member countries.[14c] There were five major criteria studied: 1) spending per capita and spending as a percentage of GDP; 2) infant mortality; 3) life expectancy; 4) fairness of financial contributions; and 5) responsiveness of system.

Not only does the United States spend by far the most per capita and the most as a percentage of GDP, but our infant mortality rate of 7.2 (per 1,000 live births) was only fourteenth best out of the top 29 countries that make up the Organization for Economic Cooperation and Development (OECD). The OECD members are considered the most industrialized advanced nations in the world. The eleven major European countries, Canada, and Australia, all did better than the United States. (Some argue this is misleading, since our infant mortality for whites is only 6.0, which would tie us for the lead with the United Kingdom. But our rate is 7.2 because the infant mortality among our black population is a dismal 14.3!)

Our disability adjusted life expectancy (DALE) at 70 years ranked 24th out of 29. Our rank on fairness of financial contribution (FFC), which is a measure of how evenly the cost burden of the system is distributed across the population, was 55th, by far the worst of any developed nation on the planet.

Finally, remarkably, the United States ranked the best in the world on "responsiveness," a measure of how well caregivers were at meeting the needs of the individual patient and treating them with respect and dignity. Of course this ranking is a bit tainted by the fact that 15% of our population really has little access to the system in the first place, so they just might have a hard time finding any caregiver, responsive or not!

# Disrobe Completely

The WHO also measured overall "attainment" based on the five criteria above and overall "performance" given its level of resources. The United States ranked 15th on attainment and an astonishing 37th for performance!

Interestingly, while overall "satisfaction" with the system in the United States was 40% (i.e. 40% reported being satisfied with our health care system), only Italy ranked worse at 20% among the 29 OECD nations.

So, this is not the kind of report card we would like to have if in fact we are the envy of the world! What remains true is that our system offers some of the best trained caregivers, the best equipped hospitals, and the most advanced approaches technologically of any of the countries of the world. It would seem that the availability and cost of these services are where are five problem areas rear their ugly heads.

Let's look at these five major areas of concern briefly.

## Insurance

First, insurance. Who are we kidding, here? In 1995 over 85% of claims filed were for less than $100! That has only risen to $200 in 2006. We now expect insurance companies to pay for everything, including routine preventative care. I can promise you that in the immediate post-war (WWII) period, when companies first began offering health benefits in lieu of higher salaries for all sorts of tax reasons, they did not envision the Frankenstein's monster to which they gave birth.

The insurance industry drives health care costs skyward in two basic ways. One is obvious—the other not so blatant. The first of course, is profit. For instance, the market capitalization, or total stock value of the American HMO industry rose from $3 billion in 1987 to almost $39 billion in 1997. During this twelve-fold increase, the United States stock market as a whole rose a little less than four fold![15] Hey, this is America. I don't begrudge them a profit. Bidness is bidness! But when you ask the average American to give you a dollar figure for his annual health care costs, what does he give you? Not the *actual* cost, but the *insurance premiums* he pays. Well—news flash—that ain't the cost! United States citizens spent $5,267 per capita for health care in 2002. That is the total estimate of expenditure on health care divided by the number of citizens. That's 53% more than the per capita rate of Germany, the next closest nation in the world.[16] Secondly, the insurance industry pushes costs up inadvertently by decoupling actual health care costs from the patient's pocketbook. All of us know that if you've met your deductible and you show up in the ER with a migraine and they say, "Maybe we ought to do an MRI scan for $1,400," you say, "Go for it!"

As we shall see in more detail, as traditional indemnity plans are supplanted by preferred provider organizations (PPOs) and, more recently, multiple variations of health maintenance organizations (HMOs), deductibles have been greatly reduced or even eliminated for in-network care, with the patient paying only a token co-pay at the point of service. So insurance companies increase costs in the whole system directly by increasing premiums to maintain profit and indirectly by inadvertently encouraging user-ship with low co-pays.

As of January 1995, the nation's four largest HMOs posted liquid assets of greater than $1 billion apiece. As of December 1994, according to *The Wall Street Journal*, six mid-sized HMOs were sitting on roughly $500 million dollars each in cash. These liquid assets accrued at greater than 15% for many HMO firms in fiscal 1994. Wall street analysts were kept busy just trying to guess where the giants would put their excess cash next! The incredible money to be made fostered the lightning-fast increase of "for-profit" HMOs over the "non-profit," traditional hospital model. From 1981 to 1998, "for-profit" HMOs went from having 12% of enrollees to 63% and from 18% of plans to 74% by 1998.[17] Currently over 90% of HMO plans are run by "for-profit" corporations. (Compared, for instance, to only 13% of community hospitals registered as "for-profit" entities.)

But increased user-ship increases total health care costs, and that may damage HMO profits even as it enlarges their number of enrollees. After phenomenal growth in the early 1990s, user-ship started to eat up many HMOs, and overall industry profitability dropped sharply starting in late 1995. This was reflected with an average annual return on HMO stocks falling from an incredible 1988-1995 average of 38%, to the 1995-1997 average of -11%! That number continued to fall after the millennium, although in the last four years or so it has been once again on the rise. As an industry response, user-ship became subject to insurer control as well, as we have discussed earlier with respect to "gatekeepers."

As user-ship rose, HMOs continued to try to keep premiums down competitively as they wrestled with each other for market share. While in 1997, 60% of HMOs reported losing money, still enrollments rose 72% for the entire industry and revenues were up 77%. However, as "gatekeeper" models spread and the insurance industry raised premiums to their employer clients, profitability rapidly returned. HMOs raised premiums 2% in 1997, 3% in 1998, and predictions at the time have held true in that rates currently increase between 6% and 9% per year on average. In only one year, the picture was turned around, and by 1998 returns on HMO stocks were back up to an average of 7% and in general haven't looked back.[18] The public backlash by 1999 over the intrusive nature of the most restrictive HMO policies, however, has seen a generally agreed diminishment in these companies' power and influence over the marketplace. They were forced to roll back some of their most egregious gatekeeper models and rely more on discounted fee for service at contracted rates through PPOs. At the time of this writing, extremely restrictive gatekeeper models are receding as viable profit-making entities for the insurance industry.

Despite managed care's claims of promoting sweeping cost savings in the delivery of health care, these savings may often be realized primarily by the insurer themselves, not the consumer corporations who contract with them. In general, these profits are not necessarily passed on to stockholders either. For the most part, they're being used to acquire larger and larger shares of the health care market and pay outrageous executive salaries for those in the nation's largest insurance conglomerates.

# The Problem

With all its problems, the greatest insurance industry dilemma is that roughly 43 million people can't even find a way to obtain it! Paradoxically, while the insurance industry in its present form is certainly part of the problem, it's also part of the solution from the perspective of those working poor who cannot afford coverage.

## Medicare/Medicaid

Our well-meaning, socially progressive, early 60s federal government decided that it should be the sole keeper of the elderly and the downtrodden. You remember—the same government that brought you the well-oiled piece of machinery called welfare. Well, great idea, guys, but a few problems have arisen. From fraud to incompetence to under funding, coupled with poor management, to all the problems associated with any massive, top-heavy bureaucracy, Medicare/Medicaid illustrates the federal government's inability to manage an unimaginably complex social issue and unscrupulous individual's proclivity to take advantage of same. Medicare made up 19% of the $1.34 trillion in spending on personal health care in 2002, with Medicaid and state children's health-insurance programs making up 18%, other public sources 7%, out of pocket 16%, and private health-insurance 36%. In other words, public sources made up 44% of all spending!

In short, Medicare/Medicaid is a huge government program, and it is projected to grow at least 10% per year over the next ten years. Personal health spending in general continues to increase as a percentage of gross domestic product (GDP) from 7.7% in 1980 to 12.8% in 2002, the highest in the world. Medicare grew from only $33.9 billion in 1980 to $272.4 billion in 2003. Medicare's share of spending however, varies immensely with type of service. For instance, Medicare made up only 20.3% of physician compensation but 30.7% of hospital, 31.6% of home health, and 31.6% of medical equipment.[19] (In 2005, Medicare accounted for only 1.6% of prescription drug costs, but in 2006, the federal government will begin to see massive expenditures as it institutes its prescription drug coverage for seniors.)

But in the last decade, Medicare/Medicaid's contribution to rising health care costs has been directly attributable to their decreasing compensation for services. The Balanced Budget Act of 1997 passed by Congress instituted deep cuts in compensation to Medicare providers, cuts which varied tremendously depending on the branch of medicine. Some surgical specialties (like gynecology and cardiothoracic surgery) saw reimbursement for major procedures drop anywhere from 50% to 90%! In the year prior to 2000, one hundred HMOs either drastically reduced their service areas or terminated their contracts with Medicare, affecting more than 400,000 Medicare beneficiaries. The reasons cited were inadequacy of Medicare payment rates and regulatory burden of participating in Medicare at all.[20]

Some physicians are abandoning Medicare for exactly the same reasons. In my practice in 2006, only two out of five of us have decided to continue to see Medicare patients. The two of us who have elected to stay lose money with every single patient interaction, our reimbursement being considerably lower than our overhead. Nationwide across all specialties, 30% have dropped out of Medicare even though that rate stayed stable in 2004–2005 despite a 5.4% decrease in reimbursement rates from the government in 2002. Some have argued this as evidence that decreasing physician fees will not cause a decrease in access for seniors. But it should be noted that Congress raised reimbursement by about 1.5% in each of the years 2003, 2004, and 2005, effectively off-setting the earlier decrease. Many physicians argue that it is the restraints and absurd federal penalties for potential billing errors of as little as $100 which make doctors shy away from the federal program. Several well-meaning United States senators sponsored legislation which has led to penalties of a $10,000 fine and/or ten years in prison for such errors.

# The Problem

Many estimates are that less than 50% of physicians will accept Medicare within the next few years unless some drastic changes are made. Medicare is planning an additional rate decrease across ICD-9 (diagnostic) and CPT (procedure) codes in the upcoming year. A much larger proportion of primary-care physicians than specialists have stayed with Medicare, and these are the physicians who make less than $120,000 per year. Specialties that rely on cash payment such as dermatology and plastic surgery typically do not accept Medicare, and a much lower percentage than the 70% for generalists accept Medicare within both medical and surgical sub-specialties.[21]

While decreasing compensation is supposed to help lower costs, it has the opposite effect by driving cost shifting to private insurers across the board. And what do they do in turn? Bingo! Raise premiums. Where did you think the $37.50 Tylenol pill came from? Are the hospitals just gouging you? Maybe a little, but mostly not. In many states, private institutions are forced by law to care for all indigents that walk in the door, particularly if their needs are deemed "emergent." You're already paying for their health care at your neighborhood state/county facility, but many of our state legislatures, in a politically correct dedication to egalitarianism, have mandated that the indigent *have a right* to the same quality health care that you working stiffs do. As a consequence, private emergency rooms and labor and delivery units across the country are seeing increasing numbers of indigents who eschew the public-hospital systems purposefully funded and available to provide for their care. Would you wait in a county hospital's ER or clinic if you could take the train for a buck uptown and walk into the most exclusive private hospital in the area, demand care, and then receive it because the state legislature mandated it? You bet you would. In our private maternity hospital in North Dallas, we have faced many a night when indigents make up 30-40% of admissions, and our own private patients have no beds. Now, before you accuse me of being elitist or at least not politically correct, realize that you are paying for system redundancy three times over! Your federal Medicare and income taxes support your county facility and provide for the indigent. Your state income, sales and property taxes support your public facilities and provide for the indigent. Your increased premiums due to your private hospital's necessary cost shifting provides for the indigent as well in terms of access!

If we as a society decide that health care is a *right* and not a *goal*, then we have the *obligation* to ensure that said health care is delivered, and delivered absolutely equally. If we impose that obligation on the federal government, it will be empowered to use its sweeping authority to ensure that the right to health care is enforced equally. It can and will tax you without recourse; it can and will require any confidential information it sees fit; it can and will regulate any facet of the medical-industrial complex; it can and will determine which approved plan you may participate in; and it *can and will* decide who you may choose as your doctor.

I submit that, despite our benevolent intent as members of society to provide for the less fortunate, *sophisticated health care is not a legal right but a privilege.* We may strive through private charity, through personal voluntarism, through our organized religious outlets, even through some government entitlement, to provide *basic* health care for the less fortunate. But to declare all forms of health care a *right* mandates absolute equality of deliverance and eliminates the role of the very same free market forces that built our current system into the envy of the world. Still, we must provide access to basic health care not only for indigents but for the working poor who make too much for Medicaid but still far too little to afford any type of insurance. Our current lack of access for these hard-working people should be a source of international embarrassment and is morally reprehensible.

The single-party payor system, i.e. the federal government as insurer, has been proposed to meet this obligation. Many other forms of government-controlled managed competition have been set forth as well. But even without any of these changes, recall that you currently get to pay three times for health care! You pay with federal taxes for Medicaid/Medicare, state and local taxes for county facilities, and you pay for higher insurance premiums brought on by the aforementioned laws guaranteeing indigent care at private facilities, coupled with decreasing Medicare/Medicaid payouts which further drive cost shifting. Remember also that should health care become federalized, the bottom line will come into focus as paramount in ways the public can't even imagine. Take this occurrence as an example. A large American tobacco company was forced in the late 1990s to provide education and advertising dollars for a campaign to discourage teenage smoking. This was the first time in history that a corporation was permitted by a government to continue selling its product while required to actively undermine its future market. But the interesting stuff comes up when we see what happened in Europe, where the majority of health care is socialized or federally funded. The Germans actually refused to allow the tobacco manufacturer's ad campaign to run on television and in print within their borders. Why? Because the state's health budget was *dependent* on a certain average life expectancy. If large numbers of youth stopped smoking, too many people would live into old age in the future and potentially bankrupt their system! Hmmm. A federal government making health care decisions for its population with the bottom line in mind . . . interesting thought.

## Defensive Medicine & Liability Crisis

Number three on the hit parade is defensive medicine. The Clinton administration offered $35 billion as an annual estimate for excess cost related to civil litigation, with $6 billion of that related specifically to defensive medicine. The AMA estimated well over $75 billion, a number I feel to be much closer to the truth. In fact, any number you pick is probably low. In 2006, the estimate was more than twice that amount. The debate continues to rage about what constitutes a crisis and whether or not one even really exists. The Public Law Research Institute at University of California's Hastings College of Law published a 1995 review of the costs of litigation, concluding that it was all blown out of proportion and based largely on the media and the public's misperception of reality. "Public perception of our legal system is clouded with myths and half truths. These misperceptions contribute to the notion that there has been a general litigation explosion. In reality there has been no litigation explosion."[22]

The author, Than Luu, claims that only a tiny subset of cases with high stakes or extended processing times have reported exorbitant legal costs.

Well, that's interesting. Note that the PLRI is doing what many law schools do when discussing the liability "crisis." They are equating costs of civil litigation with the amount of money paid to law firms on opposing sides. As we have already noted, that hardly scratches the surface of the actual cost to society. There is lost productivity from the litigants, there is the payout of the settlement or judgment, and as we physicians know on a personal basis, there is the rising cost of insurance premiums . . . insurance which, by the way, is *mandated* by state law and hospital bylaws for staff. A study by Duke University tried to quantify the huge loss represented by our current medical-legal tort system to society as a whole. "Benefits" represented malpractice (or patient injury) deterred by the threat of litigation, while "costs" represented actual dollar values spent. Their extensive and detailed research concluded that "the overall expected cost of the medical tort system in 2002 was $113.7 billion, while the expected benefits are $33.0 billion."[23]

Here's why I think there might be a teeny-weenie little "crisis," at least in the medical field:

- The median jury award in medical liability cases has doubled from 1997 to 2003, increasing from $157,000 to $300,000, with the average jury award increasing from $347,134 to $430,727.

# The Problem

- Settlement amounts reflect the above, increasing from a median of $100,000 to $200,000 and an average of $212,861 to $322,544.

- Losses due to medical liability claims are the primary driver of increases in insurance premiums, according to the federal government's general accounting office.*

- There are 125,000 active medical malpractice suits against physicians in the United States on any given day—a number just over twice the number of current medical students at all levels combined.

- Even though 75% of medical liability claims were closed without payment to the plaintiff in 2003, costs to defendants still averaged $17,408. In cases that went to trial but the defense won, costs jumped to $87,720 .[24]

- The average Ob/Gyn is now estimated to spend over 35% of his *gross* income on insurance premiums!

- As physicians are being driven out of practice, out of certain specialties, or out of certain geographic areas, patients will find it harder and harder to obtain care.

- Emergency rooms are losing staff and scaling back trauma units. Many Ob/Gyns and family practitioners have stopped delivering babies, and some high-risk procedures are being postponed by patients who cannot find a surgeon to perform them.


Witness the following statistics:

- Serious patient-access issues exist in at least twenty crisis states, with twenty-four more states nearing crisis at the end of 2004.

- One in seven Ob/Gyns was no longer delivering babies by June of 2004. (Estimates in 2006 are closer to 1 in 5.)

- 56% of Blue Cross/Blue Shield plans in crisis states report that physicians are leaving their practices, leaving their state, retiring, or abandoning higher-risk procedures.

- 45% of all hospitals report a reduction in emergency-room coverage and loss of physicians.

- 82% of Americans believe that physicians are being forced to leave their practices due to excessive litigation and the high cost of insurance premiums.

- 48% of American medical students report that liability issues are a factor in their choice of medical specialty.[25]

- The AMA Report on the Medical Liability Crisis from February 2005 goes on to point out that it is the patient who bears the ultimate cost of the crisis. Enacting certain federal reforms could result in huge savings for the entire nation's economy.

- The Congressional Budget Office (CBO) estimates that direct spending just for federal health-insurance programs (like Medicare) would be reduced by $14.9 billion over ten years with liability reform (CBO est. of HR 5, the Health Act, 2003).

- The Office of Technology Assessment (OTA) estimated over $50 billion would be saved with minimal tort reform; this dovetailed with the landmark study of the topic by Kessler and McClellen.[26]

- CBO further estimated an additional $6 billion saved by state and local governments due to reduced premiums for insurance they provide their employees.

- Huge indirect costs are laid on the health care system from the current liability situation. Defensive medicine includes any tests and treatments performed to help prevent lawsuits rather than specifically for the health of the patients. The cost of these actions is controversial and difficult to measure, but the United States Department of Health and Human Services estimate in March of 2003 was from $70 to $126 billion annually. (Note: studies like that of Andersen and Hussey in *Health Affairs*, Vol. 24, Issue 4, pp. 903–914, quote only the cost of "defending U.S. malpractice claims" at $6.5 billion or 0.46% of United States health care spending. But this represents only legal fees and grossly misrepresents what is meant by the "cost of defensive medicine," which includes tests and treatments out of fear of litigation, as well as costs in insurance premiums and decreasing availability of services.)

- Litigation itself, including effects of defensive medicine, liability premiums, risk management, outsized awards, and legal costs accounted for 7% of the total in insurance premiums (Pricewaterhouse Coopers Study, April 2002).[27]

Let's go back to your post-deductible migraine headache. When the doc offers you an MRI or CAT scan *after* your normal neurologic and fundoscopic (eye) exam corroborated by your normal blood pressure, is he doing it because he has nothing else to offer? No. Prior to about 1978, he would offer you calm reassurance, two Percodan (pain pills), and tell you to call him in the morning if you did not feel better. And you know what? You would have left happy and cared for and a whole lot sooner than you would leave today.

Today, however, the ER doc has to consider the one in a gazillion chance that you have a brain tumor, aneurysm, sub-dural hematoma, etc. Because, God forbid, if you did have one of those and he missed it, it could cost him his career, retirement, children's education, life savings, self-esteem, little things like that. Don't get me wrong. I'm not suggesting that he shouldn't look for those things eventually, *if symptoms persist*; just that he doesn't have to look right then and there, when you may never have symptoms again!

Defensive medicine is now so ingrained that it's literally a bad habit. Doctors don't even realize it when they're doing it. Most doctors admit it and a few don't, but all physicians in the United States practice defensive medicine every minute whether they know it or not! (For an excellent review of the topic, see Dr. Richard Andersen's *Billions for Defense: The Pervasive Nature of Defensive Medicine, Archives of Internal Medicine*, Vol. 159, Nov. 8, 1999, pp. 2399–2402.) Take preoperative lab work. Often hundreds and thousands of dollars are spent on testing to uncover incredibly rare abnormalities that might lead to potential problems with the anesthetic or surgery, most of which could be handled at the time if, in fact, the near mythical problem ever actually unfolded. In short, in healthy people under fifty, preoperative bloodwork is almost always done and almost never indicated.

Other societies from Western Europe to Japan are flabbergasted at the percentage of GNP we pour down the drain for defensive medicine, for insurance to cover product liability, and for product modification to avoid problems that were once avoided by good parenting! *Wake up, America! Tort reform on a national scale is long, long overdue.*

## New Technology

The fourth big contender propelling medical costs skyward is clearly new technology. Couple this with defensive medicine along with competing hospitals in the same geographic area, and you have the prescription for logarithmic cost increases.

There is much validity to the belief that humanity has progressed more technologically in the last twenty years than it has in the preceding 80,000! Digitalized, base two, instantaneous information transfer coupled with the millions of intricate pathway options provided by interlinked computer chips has quite literally changed our world. Advances in laser technology, fiber optics, and robotics have given us further modalities with which to apply the awesome power of our computers. While MRI may allow imaging quality never before possible, and Gamma knife may allow neurosurgery without an incision, the technologies involved are quite disparate. There is one similarity though. They're expensive. Big time expensive! Millions of the little green guys! And if hospital A wants to take patients from hospital B, which happens to have a new MRI located only three miles away, they may feel they have to have their own MRI or else lose the revenue those patients will generate. Well, the General Electrics of this world didn't just fall off the turnip truck, so they *raise* their prices in this scenario, not *lower* them. Thus competition for high tech drives costs *up*, not down. If there were ten different companies making MRI machines, that might be different; but there aren't!

Where does the hospital get this kind of huge revenue? Why, from cost shifting of course! Who pays for that? You do, via increased premiums. The need for expensive equipment and procedures, remember, is not just driven by hospital competition but by defensive medicine practices as well. Thus the pressure to have the most advanced capabilities is intense, and your bill (read: your insurer's bill) will reflect it.

We should also note that technology has increased costs in a more subtle way—through the proliferation of specialists. In the 1930s only 20% of physicians were considered specialists. Insurance paid only for hospital care, and specialists required higher out-of-pocket payment than general practitioners. In the 1940s, specialists were given higher rank and higher salaries by the military. Many GPs then sought specialty training under the GI bill. In the 1950s, with federal grants for research on the rise, most were going to specialists who then dominated evolving medical schools. By 1969, 50% of doctors were specialty boarded. By 1990, 66% were specialists, and only 14% of medical students were entering primary-care residencies.[28]

So historically, better pay fueled the natural tendency to specialize in a society where the medical-legal environment demanded perfection, and the average student couldn't possibly keep pace with the technological advances in every field of medicine.

## Inflation

Lastly, there's our old friend inflation. So now it's only 4%, big deal! Now figure out what 4% of 150,000,000,000 is. I'll tell ya, it's a bunch—$4,500,000,000 or $4.5 billion. That's inflation's contribution annually to our estimate of defensive medicine costs. Ouch! Remember we spend 13% of our GDP on health care, or $1.4 trillion per year. Just 4% of THAT is right about $56 billion of additonal cost each year! As Harry Truman once said, "A billion here, a billion there, and pretty soon you're talking about real money!"

# The Solution: Managed Competition?

Contrary to popular belief, understanding managed competition is not humanly possible. You might as well spend time reading some recreational physics like "string theory" and how it unites the theories of gravitation, strong force, weak force, and electromagnetic force . . . good luck. "Managed competition" may be defined, as we did earlier, as a health care delivery system wherein decisions about diagnosis and treatment are made not by the people trained to do so but by people working for-profit-motivated corporations. It is a term which encompasses a myriad of paradigms for the entire medico-industrial complex, many of which have very little similarity to each other. But one thing is clear, managed competition involves a radical departure from our current system of third-party payors, free choice of doctor and facility, and government care of the indigent through county facilities funded by Medicaid.

There is a common thread, however. Most of the scenarios involve the insurance companies becoming the provider themselves, either by owning hospital systems and the affiliated physicians' practices or by controlling delivery through a "capitated" system where the insurer pays a group of physicians or a hospital-run corporation a certain number of dollars per patient (employee) per month for any and all care provided (i.e., per capita). The physicians are then compensated from the pool of money left over at the end of each fiscal quarter. Most of these scenarios call for "gatekeeper," primary-care physicians as described earlier. Well, guess what? Do you think this primary-care provider (family practice, internist, pediatrician)-driven system is going to allow referrals to specialists for many problems? For any problems? Not when it costs them their livelihood.

# Disrobe Completely

The doctors will be given a strong financial incentive with a capitated system to avoid expensive tests and referrals because those tests and referrals would diminish their personal income. Well, you say, that's the idea, right? We want to cut costs, don't we? No, remember the goal—we want to cut costs, increase access, and *maintain quality health care*. The assumption that the specialists we've trained over the last thirty years are now superfluous is patently absurd! Medicine has become so complex and changes so rapidly that it's difficult to keep up with your own area of expertise from week to week, much less everyone else's area as well! There is no way that quality of care can remain unaltered if the least trained physicians (in terms of years of residency) in our system are suddenly called upon to diagnose and treat conditions for which they may have little or no training. Under a capitated system of managed care, you will get a very different health care product—don't kid yourself.

Initially, when HMOs further decoupled health care costs from the consumer's pocketbook with only small co-pays at the point of service, user-ship skyrocketed. But many fledgling HMOs have failed because a co-pay of five to ten dollars, or even nothing, gives the patient no disincentive whatsoever to go to the doctor for the slightest problem. As user-ship rose, so did costs. But many managed care companies and their parent insurers have found new ways to counter this trend by actually limiting number of visits permitted per year, whether to emergency rooms, primary providers, or specialists.

For instance, I have a friend and patient who has a rare form of multiple sclerosis. She is a wife and mother of two, and without an expensive, rarely used medicine delivered intravenously every few months, she becomes completely paralyzed to the point of mechanical ventilation several times already. Not only will her insurer not pay for this "experimental drug," which is the only one that can help her, but they *limit* the total number of visits she can have to health care providers per year. In her case, by late spring of each year, her insurer no longer pays for the visits to any of her physicians, nor even to the physical therapy which is ongoing and deemed absolutely necessary for her survival. She and her husband faithfully paid premiums for over twenty years. Too bad—doesn't carry any weight with her insurer! Now they are out of money. They've used all the money they had saved for the kids' educations on the medicine she requires. There are literally thousands of such stories, of course, but it illustrates the point. Insurers know how to protect their assets. It's business.

As alluded to already, each of the nation's top ten HMOs has liquid assets estimated between $500 million and 6 billion. Many HMOs have financial positions so strong that the insurance boards of several states are beginning to question and sometimes deny rate increases. (By 2006, some estimates for the top ten HMOs place assets at over $5 billion apiece.)

Doctors and hospitals are being squeezed by HMOs to do their jobs more cheaply or risk losing portions of their patient population. And as they do their jobs more cheaply, HMOs literally have so much cash that they don't know what to do with it. HMOs in general do not provide for, or own, the medical infrastructure; thus their overhead—primarily administrative, legal and advertising costs—is low. No wonder *The Wall Street Journal* dubbed these HMO's "money machines" in December of 1994.

It would be false to imply that all the changes wrought by managed care have been negative. Companies like Columbia/HCA Health-care with its 308 hospitals and 125 outpatient facilities nationwide have forced efficiency on competing hospitals.[29] Not unlike Wal-Mart in its phenomenal growth spurred by cost-cutting efficiency, Columbia/HCA is literally calling the shots in many areas. Their ability to buy fixed overhead items in bulk allows them to consistently underbid area competitors for HMO contracts. Many of their competitors have had no choice than to become leaner. Often this means forming alliances with area facilities that used to be considered competitors or face absorption or even closure.

# Disrobe Completely

Columbia has also made innovative moves like installing computer software that improves physician efficiency by automating lab results, patient databases, and pharmaceutical information.

Nevertheless, this rising giant represents the epitome of corporate medicine. While its leadership favors tort reform and eliminating preexisting conditions, it sees no place for the nonprofit community hospital. Its hospitals are under corporate chain of command, and when the word comes down from on high, that's the way it is. The traditional board of trustees made of community-minded philanthropists has no real place in this system. Like it or not, beneficent or not, efficient or not, corporate medicine's goal is to improve the bottom line.

Assets for Columbia/HCA rose from $200 million in 1991 to $15 billion in 1994, or roughly 75 fold![30] It's a given that their profits continue to rise as well. That's great for the stockholders, probably good for the economy, but will only be good for the patient if the ability to choose her own physician is preserved and the physician is allowed to determine the course of her care. Such growth based on efficiency would be expected to pass savings on to businesses.

In fact, managed care *did* significantly reduce health care costs for many large corporations. According to a survey by the employee benefits consulting firm Foster Higgins of over 2,400 employers, over a third were able to halt or reduce their company's rising health benefits tab in fiscal 1993. They did so by putting the squeeze on doctors and hospitals. They provided financial incentive to steer employees into restrictive managed care plans and used their leverage to gain price concessions in a competitive marketplace.[31] Unfortunately for them, ever-increasing premiums and expanding lists of pensioners have gone on to destroy many of these companies' brief health care savings in the 1990s. In any event, those savings were achieved at the direct expense of the quality of health care and the patient's freedom to choose in my opinion.

Xerox contracted with 204 HMOs nationwide in 1993. Employees were given the option of traditional indemnity coverage at much higher rates, and only about 30% chose to make the financial sacrifice necessary to maintain their freedom of choice. The other 70% of employees were given choices between different HMOs, thus forcing the HMOs to compete for Xerox premium dollars.[32] In 2004, Xerox joined with Sears, Sprint, Texas Instruments, and J.C. Penney among others, to institute care-focused purchasing (CFP). This is an attempt to use an industry-developed score-card to rate providers on cost effectiveness and "quality" scale and publish it, not unlike *Consumer Reports* for consumer products. Mercer Corp. is offering the plan to large employers and says the "quality" standards come from the nonprofit regulatory agencies—the National Committee on Quality Assurance (NCQA) and the Joint Commission on Accreditation of Health-care Organizations (JCAH).[32a]

In all honesty, these organizations are not viewed too kindly by those who actually practice medicine. The standards they create are often felt to have been created by those "not in the trenches" and tend to lead to mountains of paperwork. For example, the average hospital chart has increased in page number by a factor of more than tenfold in the last fifteen years. Each page represents time away from patient contact for the health care worker.

GTE admitted in the mid-1990s that they would like to force their 94,000 United States employees into even more restrictive plans. As it was, they kept their rate increase on the average health benefits plan to only 1% in 1993, versus the national average of 8%.

The fastest growing type of plan however, is now the "opt-out" plan where employees are given the option to pay more out-of-pocket to retain their choice of physician. DuPont's long-term strategy includes such plans for its 66,000 employees and 75,000 retirees.

At the end of 1993, 27% of employees nationwide were in a PPO plan allowing some degree of choice, 19% were in restrictive HMO "gatekeeper" plans, and 7% were in "opt-out" combinations. The remaining 47% were in some type of more traditional indemnity plan.[33]

# Disrobe Completely

At the end of 2004, public outcry and subsequent corporate pressure has severely limited the number of pure gatekeeper HMOs, but still only 4% of employees were in some type of traditional indemnity plan, down from the 47% mentioned above. The rest are all in some form of HMO, PPO, or POS. Only a tiny number are in health savings accounts or some sort.

Despite these "improvements" in the cost of care realized in the mid-1990s, by the year 2005, with roughly 96% of benefits offered in the form of some managed care, health care benefits were by far the most rapidly rising overhead for all companies who offered them. Even though costs were held down briefly in the 1990s, they are now rising at the alarming rate of 14% per year, with rising managed care premiums hobbling thousands of companies. For larger companies such as airlines, automobile manufacturers, railroads, and hotel chains, health benefit increases demanded by employee unions and by pensioners were one of the most frequent causes of catastrophic financial failure, such as Chapter 11 bankruptcy.

So, all forms of managed competition will tend to provide "less" medicine with respect to possibly needed tests and referrals and will be forced to combat higher user-ship with restrictions on access. It seems clear that managed care did briefly lower the cost of health care or at least slowed its rise in some circumstances in the nineties. But does it now maintain the quality which we agreed at the outset was the other portion of our goal for reform? Is that "quality" quantifiable in a way that employers as purchasers of health care can really use? Even if companies shell out millions to consultants to evaluate length of stay, referral patterns, mortality rates, prescribing patterns, test fees, and office-visit charges, can they accurately assess, for example, the feeling a woman needs to have about her Ob/Gyn right before she climbs into the stirrups for a very personal problem? Can they *accurately assess the value* of the extra phone call at home to check on her after her surgery, or the hand held tightly while she goes to sleep knowing you'll take good care of her during her operation, or the kind of relationship

# The Solution: Managed Competition?

where a hug is natural and a true comfort in the face of bad news?

The vice president of marketing for one of the fastest growing insurance providers in Texas said in an interview recently, "What they [the public] perceive as high quality is not really quality at all." The implication is that Aetna, MetLife, Sanus, Prucare, Cigna, Humana, etc., know what is high quality, and in their paternalistic beneficence, will make those decisions for you.[34] Already insurers are eliminating or "de-selecting" the physicians who cost them the most money. The ones who remain on their network will be the ones who deliver the cheapest health care. The definition of "quality" used to be the care that led to the best outcome. Not anymore. The vice president of health services management for a large Texas insurer has said that "quality medicine *is cost-effective medicine*."[35] Evidently the old adage, "You get what you pay for," applies in all walks of life except medicine.

Proponents of managed care say that the new managed care systems will impose discipline on physicians who were formerly guided by only their own avarice. The exact opposite is actually the case. The autonomous private physician makes referrals, orders CAT scans, etc., when he deems them appropriate. There is no financial incentive for these decisions except for the few who abuse lab ownership, which has largely been curtailed by Congress's Stark legislation. On the contrary, the HMO physician must allow finances to play a major role in his decisions. Under the new paradigm, every diagnostic test, every referral, every expensive treatment adversely affects his personal income!

In most insurance-owned HMO systems, the managed care company contracts directly with the employer, and then the HMO contracts with providers such as hospitals, surgi-centers, and physicians. Who has the motivation to meet the patients' needs? The hospital strives to please its customer, the HMO; the HMO wants only to please its customer, the corporate employer, and of course its own shareholders. Again, who wants to please the patient? If the physician has large portions of his patients contracted from the HMO, or worse, if he has an exclusive arrangement, where must he place his first allegiance? When the interests of the HMO and those of the individual patient clash, how will the contract physician prioritize? To be honest, PPOs are not that different. The insurer who offers a PPO plan contracts directly with the hospital or surgi-center with fixed payments for services and length of stay. They also contract with the physician at discounted rates for every service provided. Physicians can be dropped from PPO lists just as they can be from HMOs. When the physician is faced with "de-selection," the very loss of his patients, for practice not deemed adequately cost-effective by the insurer, will his decisions not be tainted? Who then is motivated to put the needs of the patient above all else? The answer is simple and regrettable. The answer is *no one.*

Managed competition succeeds in devaluing the physician-patient relationship to near nonexistence. Don't delude yourself when you hear different systems promise you "choice." They mean you may select from a limited list of providers with which they have contracted. In fact, employers in the last several years are being encouraged by health care thinktanks to utilize "select [narrow] networks" in which an even smaller subset of providers within an insurer's network have agreed to work for even less compensation. Employees are steered toward these subselect networks in exchange for paying a smaller portion of the premium or having a lower deductible or any number of approaches. The same strategy is employed to steer employees' choices of physician and usage of specialists. These contracts are never for more than a year, so you could be forced to change providers annually. Already we see patients who have been with our practice for ten years, who develop a condition requiring surgery (i.e., major hospital expense), and they're forced to seek another physician and hospital if we're no longer on their network.

Who cares, you might ask? You may forget that physicians are people too. I may strive to give the same care to everyone who crosses the threshold to my office, but I know it doesn't happen. If I've delivered all four of a woman's chil-

# The Solution: Managed Competition?

dren and feel a part of their family, I go to extraordinary efforts to keep them happy and well. Not to mention that the patient's comfort level with her physician dictates her openness and willingness to provide an accurate history of what might be an intimate or embarrassing problem. Medical history is still 95% of the diagnostic process, and an inadequate history because of patient discomfort or time constraints leads to errors in judgment.

So, managed competition might decrease some costs for some time, but won't appreciably increase access, grossly restricts the patient's own authority to make choices for themselves, decreases the level of care in terms of technology and expertise, and undermines the physician-patient relationship.

## Some Answers

Why not nationalize health care? You could probably write another entire book in an effort to answer this question. But many people are so fed up with spiraling costs, lack of access for millions, the incredible complexity of even trying to understand a statement from their insurer, that the "simplicity" of a one party payor starts to look attractive even to physicians. At the end of another endless day of haggling with insurers, Medicare, JCAH, OSHA etc., watching patients move on to other doctors and hospitals because of job and benefit changes, dealing with the frustration of therapies or diagnoses denied; well then it starts to seem like it couldn't be any worse. But it could.

As mentioned 45% of all health care dollars spent in the country are public already and look at the mess we have currently. You need look no further than the defense department budget if you really believe the federal government will run "health care" efficiently. You may think that one payor means that with everyone essentially on the same insurance, that there will be no limitation of choice, but the exact opposite looms. The Federal government will not be letting you see a specialist when YOU think you need to but when THEY think you need to. The gross restrictions of the mid '90s HMOs will become institutionalized within the federal health care system.

Furthermore, it flies in the face of free enterprise from every single standpoint whether you are a physician, hospital, pharmaceutical company, or biotechnical company. The alteration of incentive created will almost assure that the best and brightest will no longer seek a career in medicine or the allied fields. Medicine will dumb down to the same extent that the public school system has.

And what of the government's motives on a day-to-day basis? Will the bureaucrats in Washington have much of a motivation or any kind of ability to deal with you personally even though they'll be calling the shots? Think you'll get a lot of personal attention when you are one of 300 million? Remember the story of big tobacco in Germany a few years ago. The government refused to allow anti-smoking commercials on the air because it might *decrease* the death rate which would be catastrophic for the nation's socialized economy! The Germans depend on a certain number of people dying of cancer and heart disease annually in order to budget for care of the elderly. In short, decisions will be made once nationalized on the greater good, not necessarily as you see it, but as the less than a thousand people or so in the District of Columbia see it.

No, national health care is not the answer to the desire for "universal health care." We can achieve universal access by addressing each of the problem areas we have outlined without destroying the heart of the system that has, until very recently, been the envy of the world.

As previously intimated, neither I nor anyone else has the answers on how to put out the firestorm of controversy surrounding health care in this country. But many of us have suggestions about how to at least avoid suffocating in the foam from our own extinguishers! There are now a myriad of consulting corporations which you can easily locate on the Web who propose all sorts of solutions, at least for the employers' dilemma of costs rising out of control. But below are some thoughts pertaining to only our big five issues behind the crisis.

# The Solution: Managed Competition?

## Insurance

First, we must restore the link between actual costs and patient payment. If a third party pays the bill for anything, you're going to buy more than if you're footing it yourself. There have been many proposals about how to deal with this phenomenon. I believe the most logical would include medical IRAs or so-called medical savings accounts (MSAs) offered by employers or, alternately, the government. If it is true that the average annual cost of health care to a family of four is less than $1,500, then something close to this amount could be withheld (approximately $120/month) and placed in an interest-bearing investment account. This account would be coupled with a high-deductible, low-cost catastrophic insurance plan. Routine visits to the doctor would not involve any insurance claims or even significant paperwork, cutting down administrative cost. The charges would be handled electronically by a debit card drawing on your MSA for anything under the deductible of your medical plan. These types of plans now fall under the umbrella term "consumer-driven health plans" (CDHPs) with the older term "medical savings account" being replaced by health care reimbursement accounts (HRAs) or health care spending accounts (HSAs). Effective January 1, 2004, the federal government has allowed the creation of multiple plans which operate along these lines, allowing the money which is set aside and unused to roll over to the next year and thus accumulate. Money used for qualifying health purposes is then tax free and accumulates tax free. HRAs and HSAs are technically available to 250 million Americans under retirement age. "Archer" MSAs are available to self-employed individuals or companies who have less than fifty-one employees on average in either of the previous two years. The money set aside may be funded entirely by the employer or entirely by the employee or anywhere in between, depending on what the employer chooses to offer.

# Disrobe Completely

Funding for the HSAs would come from savings generated by switching to low-cost/high-deductible policies or from employer contributions. Catastrophic costs, such as surgeries for illness or accidents, would be handled with traditional insurance provided by the employer via a traditional insurance carrier but at a theoretically less expensive rate for, say, a $5,000–$10,000 deductible policy. (Currently a family of four may pay $600 to $900 per month to their insurer [or their employer pays this or a portion of this amount] or approximately $7,200 to $10,800 per year for a traditional HMO or PPO with a lower deductible. If average actual health costs are truly about $1,500 per year, three guesses at who keeps the profit! If you guessed the insurer, then you win!)

Unfortunately, the insurance industry really has control of the possibility of success for HSAs because it controls the premium charged for the attached high-deductible catastrophic plan. In our small office in Dallas (38 employees), for example, the best offer we could find on an HSA offered by a major insurance carrier was an $890/month premium for a $10,000 deductible policy coupled with $400/month additional contribution to the savings portion of the HSA! In other words, $1,290/month for the privalege of a $10,000 deductible! Now, you and I both know who's getting rich on this deal. Even so, the savings do accrue tax free and may be accessed simply with a debit card to your account with no hassle whatsoever. Many may choose to pay the price just for the convenience, lack of hassle, rapid completion of transactions, and freedom to choose wherever you wish to spend the health care dollar. Of course there is yet another hidden catch . . . if you spend your HSA dollar on a provider who is not in the catastrophic insurer's network, it may well be applied to a separate and *even higher out-of-network deductible!*

Americans want the best buy for their money. If the ER doc says there's very little chance of a serious underlying cause to your headache, then you'll be willing to take the two Percodan and call him in the morning, potentially averting the $1,400 charge that would have come out of your own account. Of course, he may not offer you that option openly, without tort reform!

# The Solution: Managed Competition?

## Advantages Of HSAs

There are many potential advantages to a reform package centered on HSAs. The Private Medical Foundation of Shawnee, Oklahoma, points out the following eight:

1. Saving Money: People will purchase medical care with their HSA funds and thus be better shoppers.

2. Restore the doctor-patient relationship: The two individuals most concerned about an individual health problem work together to fix it without a bureaucrat or insurance company employee to guide them.

3. Maintain the Quality of Care: HSAs would allow the health caremarketplace to self-correct through free choice. The patient and physician together would choose the best course of action tailored individually to that case, not as "allowed" by a third party whose only concern is profit.

4. Encourage Rationing by Choice: Families and individuals would decide which monies would be spent on health care and which on other essentials.

5. Provide funds for Preventive Care: HSAs would be available for preventive exams and testing often not covered by insurance.

6. Provide for Insurance Premiums: HSAs accrued over time would provide for premiums during periods of unemployment.

7. Long-Term Care: HSA funds not expended during working years would be available for Medicare supplement over age sixty-five.

8. Benefits Personal and Portable: HSAs would be private personal property and would go with the employee when jobs changed.[36]

# Disrobe Completely

If HSAs or their equivalent have not been mentioned by your employer, inquire further. If you choose a managed care plan instead, encourage your benefits personnel to avoid "gatekeeper," insurance-owned systems at all costs. These systems are the most restrictive with respect to both patient choice and physician authority and luckily are dying out as of 2006. Instead, your employer might seek out physician-owned, physician-run, multi-specialty groups. While these groups may function on a "capitated" basis, they often avoid "gatekeeping" in the recognition that it fosters substandard care. Medical decisions with respect to quality assurance, outcome data, diagnostic and therapeutic cost efficiencies are at least made by the ones who have the knowledge to make them rather than para-medical financial personnel.

In short, even for the self-employed or small-company employee, an HSA offers a way to cover routine health care expenses, linking the actual costs to the patient's pocket but allowing the individual to accumulate money tax-free in a rollover investment account similar to an IRA. A portion of the money set aside would or could go toward paying the premium on a high-deductible, low-cost catastrophic policy. To be truly effective at national health care cost-cutting however, the insurers cannot be allowed to charge exhorbitant premiums for the high-deductible component! Furthermore, HSA expenses to *any* provider must be allowed to come off of the same deductible. Finally, the low-paid, blue-collar worker is extremely unlikely to benefit from this plan without significant initial and ongoing funding from his employer. Unless the employer gets behind the idea enthusiastically and with dollars, the average worker will be put off by the high-deductible which could leave him in real financial trouble with say, an unexpected hospitalization.

Other options are being explored for the low-income worker such as health care premiums as a percentage of base pay. In this initiative, higher paid employees of a corporation would pay higher premiums, and lower paid employees would pay lower premiums for the same insurance benefits package. Computerized payroll systems and departments dedicated to benefit administration can more easily implement this type of complex plan than in past years.

Pharmaceuticals are rising faster than any other segment of the health care dollar. Many employers are considering health reimbursement accounts (HRAs) for pharmacy benefits alone; mandatory mail in prescription plans for those on maintenance meds; requiring benefits managers to make employees aware on a statement of the actual price of pharmaceuticals when choices may be possible.

Huge savings may be obtained purchasing the most commonly used prescription meds overseas using the Internet. An Israeli company, for instance, can provide anti-hypertensive and cholesterol-lowering drugs at up to 70% off retail prices in America. Personally I believe there should be no legal restraints on the purchase of prescription meds for those who have actually had them prescribed. International trade agreements could be sought to either insure that meds which United States law requires be prescribed by a physician are in fact prescribed, or that alternately, pharmaceuticals be labelled clearly with respect to the dangers of using not under a physician's care. Restoring personal responsibility to our society includes a modicum of "buyer beware." The only other reason for restrictions on overseas purchase of meds is the pharmaceutical company's profit margins. I'm in favor of a for-profit drug industry, and I understand that they spend tremendous numbers of dollars on research and development. But some medicines have a ten- to a hundred-fold disparity in their price overseas vs. the United States and the consumer should at least be allowed to participate in market forces which might equalize things a bit. If we truly favor "free trade," this is a reasonable place to start.

In any event, while consumers struggle with getting affordable insurance coverage, physicians may be forced to find their own answers if the system as a whole continues to drastically decrease their compensation and severely restrict their decision-making power as well as their patients' ability to stick with them. While the FTC restricts the ability of physicians to collectively bargain with insurers, they can't keep large numbers of them from telling the insurers to jump

in a lake! Over 10% of the Ob/Gyns in the United States now refuse to participate in *any* insurance plan. Their patients must pay cash up front, and then file
with their insurer themselves. While leading currently to "carriage" practices for
the rich in some parts of the country, more and more physicians may be forced
to consider this option if compensation rates keep falling and malpractice keeps
rising. Physicians may be notoriously bad at business and bad at flying airplanes,
but most of us are at least pretty good at addition and subtraction.

## Medicaid/Medicare

But our next problem, you will recall, is Medicaid/Medicare. This one won't
be easy to fix. This behemoth must be contained by limiting the number of people
who benefit from it. Many, many working people are on Medicaid both legally
and illegally. If the blue-collar worker could afford high-deductible insurance with
a partially employer funded HSA for routine costs, he wouldn't need to be on
Medicaid. In fact, federal dollars currently directed to Medicaid could be used to
subsidize low-income workers so that their HSAs were adequately funded. This,
combined with legislation regulating catastrophic premiums such that the working poor could enter the system, should be considered a viable option.

- Perhaps affluent retirees who absolutely do not need Medicare due to
  their income levels could be suspended from benefits or asked to volun-
  tarily suspend themselves even though they were taxed for it their entire
  working lives, until such time as they could show that they do need it.
  (While we're at it, we could fix Social Security the same way. Once eligi-
  ble age is reached, those whose annual retirement income exceeded say
  $100,000, for example, could simply not receive their benefits! This level
  or any other picked by Congress could be reviewed every four years
  or so. Yes, people would have contributed taxes their entire lives for
  someone else's retirement, but making this reform would only require a
  change of mindset. If you are doing well by retirement age, then you've
  helped the less fortunate; if you're doing poorly, then the safety net is in

place. My parents will probably want to kill me for this suggestion! But hey, I have my *own* AARP card now and I'm entitled to an opinion. Or if you don't like that plan, simply increase the age at which Social Security can be withdrawn! Life expectancy has increased almost twenty years since Social Security was introduced, but the age at which benefits can be withdrawn has not been increased. That is crazy! Exactly the same logic applies for Medicare. The age for Medicare *must* be progressively increased as our population's useful working age increases. It's insane to have the same retirement age in 2006 as we had forty years ago.

- True *urban* indigents currently have access to the best doctors and technology in the world, via the state and county hospital system. Don't destroy this by decreasing funding at these levels. Shifting the care of the inner-city indigent to all private facilities via anti-dumping laws just double taxes the working public via resultant cost shifting and state and federal taxes. The working poor uninsured are often then hit the worst with private hospitals often charging full price to them rather than the 40% less that would be charged at PPO rates. Consequently those that can afford it the least are charged the most. Help the working poor not by placing them on Medicaid, but instead use those Medicaid federal dollars to help defray the cost of an HSA linked to a high-deductible catastrophic plan. Expand the county hospital systems for the care of the indigent. Support neighborhood clinics for delivery of preventive health care to this segment of the population. These are legitimate government expenditures.

- Here's an easy suggestion: allow physicians to provide pro bono services in their practices. That's right. It is now illegal for a physician to discount or no-bill a patient in his private practice! Not only are there no tax deductions allowed for donated services to charity, but Medicare regulations also make it a felony to charge different fees to Medicare and non-Medicare patients for the same services. Seems incredible but even charging "nothing" is technically a different fee scale from that charged to Medicare patients, and no variance whatsoever is allowed. That means that the federal government is standing in the way of physicians all across the nation improving access for the working poor who may well be uninsured.

- Government HSAs, or government-subsidized HSAs, and affordable catastrophic insurance may help the working poor, but the rural indigent is a different problem. True, much of the true indigent population gravitates to urban centers anyway because of the greater availability of assistance programs, public health facilities, and job opportunities. The remaining rural poor may need to be part of a Medicaid program, but one that pays reasonably for services to avoid the hidden tax to us all of cost shifting by institutions to their private patients' third-party payors. There may be a regulatory need with respect to guaranteeing rural indigents access to extensions of urban government-supported clinic systems. The income limit of $20,000 for a family to be excluded from Medicaid is simply too low. Working poor when they pass slightly above this limit still cannot afford insurance of any kind and put food on the table as well! Unless there are severe legislative restrictions placed on catastrophic insurance premiums tied to HSAs, it makes more sense to up the income limit than use this as a reason to socialize the entire system.

In any event, the current reality of managed care medicine *will* drive some of the good physicians found in urban surplus to more rural locations where they may make less money but retain higher degrees of autonomy. Some of these physicians will simply stop accepting any insurance, leaving the filing with third party payors to the patient.

## Affordable Health Care Solutions/Regional Health Care Quality Initiatives

More than fifty Fortune 500 companies have come together with a plan that gives access to affordable health-insurance for over four million of the nation's uninsured. These two coalitions are made up of more than two hundred executives at these major firms concerned about escalating costs and the drain on worker productivity. AHCS works on a national level and RHCQI on a regional level to form new alliances among employers, health care plans and providers, and hospitals and physicians within their assigned areas. The goal is to provide coverage for those working Americans currently ineligible for employer-sponsored coverage or who cannot afford individual insurance. (See www.hcpr. org/press/2004/pr_051004.asp for more info.)

While clearly in their own best interest financially, I applaud the efforts of American industry when it addresses efficiency issues whether in health care or otherwise with collective wisdom. Efforts like this one echo the elder President Bush's much maligned but heartfelt "Thousand Points of Light." Any approach to health care cost containment that does not turn to the government to solve their problem for them is in my mind what America is all about!

## Defensive Medicine

*National tort reform must be part of any legislative package for health care reform.* The entire premise of a market-force, medical-industrial complex driven solely by the legitimate costs of delivering health care depends on eliminating the direct costs of malpractice premiums and, to a much greater extent, eliminating the need for defensive medicine practices. Our young physicians are not even learning the difference between necessary testing and defensive testing. The emotional strain on practicing physicians is driving many at the peak of their medical careers to seek alternative ways to make a living. This strain develops not only from constant attention to potential legal consequences but from time and effort spent on massive piles of paperwork to file claims, acquire pre-certification for everything (always from someone not as qualified as yourself to make the decision), and hours of meetings devoted to trying to fathom the current morass of partially managed care systems.

# Disrobe Completely

Why can't plaintiff's attorneys pay the legal costs of the defendant when they lose a case? If they're so sure that malpractice was committed, surely they should be willing to bear the costs of the case if they lose. No one's asking the plaintiff's attorney to pay for the mental anguish and suffering of the unjustly accused physician and his family, but couldn't the court costs be covered, as in England and Japan?

Why can't the jury in a trial know of alternate compensation already received by the plaintiff when damages are being assessed? You know why— because the plaintiff's attorney gets a huge percentage (usually 30–40%) of the award, that's why.

So why can't the attorney work for a fee just like I do, not on contingency? Can you see your doctor telling you that if he successfully removes your kidney, he'll be taking a higher percentage of whatever we determine that kidney is worth to you?

Why is there not a cap on pain and suffering in all states instead of just a few? Does it seem right to put an arbitrary, astronomical value on an intangible thing, often in the face of no or at least already covered medical expenses? In 1994, democratic proposals before Congress actually suggested *eliminating* even the few existing caps! We should limit non economic damages to $250,000 (e.g. pain and suffering and mental anguish) nationally, as was done in Texas in 2005. It was proposed in the summer of 2006, and Congress voted it down again.

Allow no cap on true economic damages and allow punitive damages up to only $250,000 or twice the real economic damages, whichever is more.

Is joint and several liability even constitutional? Just because I am associated with an individual or institution that is culpable for actions leading to an injury, should I be held just as accountable and punished? The federal law should allocate damage awards fairly and in proportion to fault.

Should physicians be allowed a jury of their peers? If I study medicine for fifteen years, should an automotive plant worker be the one to decide on the basis of purchased expert testimony whether my actions were in error? When was it that we decided physicians aren't human and indeed are not allowed to make errors in judgment or otherwise?

According to a 2003 Gallup poll, 72% of Americans support reforms that guarantee full payment of lost wages and all medical expenses but limit non economic damages that are subjective.[37]

As mentioned earlier, detailed and extensive studies have estimated at least a $50 billion savings nationally if effective tort reform was introduced.[38] Reforms instituted in states like Texas, where non economic damages were limited to $250,000/defendant in 2005, have already led to benefits. An environment now exists where physicians in high-risk specialties are more apt to continue in practice. Malpractice premiums have stabilized and in many areas have even dropped considerably, keeping specialties like obstetrics available in rural counties, especially in the Rio Grande Valley.

## Technology

Our fourth complicating factor leading to high costs, you will recall, is the price of rapidly expanding high technology. Suppose an MRI machine costs $2 million. What do you suppose the product liability in terms of research and development, superfluous manufacturing alterations needed to protect against unreal but perceived potential threats, and direct liability insurance premiums add to the cost of that MRI? Remember the headlines in 1993: someone has already successfully litigated for the loss of their psychic ability during scanning!

The development of new pharmaceuticals and new technologies with medical applications carries some unavoidable costs. But the ten leading drug companies should not be forced overseas in part due to legal costs nearing 30% of their net income. Tort reform must include laws that ease the burden of product liability on our manufacturing sector as well as on physicians and hospitals.

# Disrobe Completely

## Inflation

Inflation is clearly beyond the exclusive control of the government in a market society. While the federal reserve can act in what it perceives to be our best interest, there is probably little we can do to deal with this aspect of rising health care costs. We can only recognize that this percentage cost annually must be taken into account to reflect the true rising cost of health care and in effect adds insult to injury. But in a similar fashion, the dollars saved with efficient reform are more valuable in an inflationary environment.

So, we have a problem. Not an insurmountable problem, for I feel short of breaching the laws of Newtonian physics, nothing is impossible for the American people. If we recognize what is good about the system, eliminate what is bad, and make sure that we don't confuse the two, we can reduce the national costs and ensure at least adequate access for all.

But if we allow the government, the insurance industry, managed competition, or anyone else to destroy the physician-patient relationship, undermine the physician's authority to make decisions, and eliminate the patients' ability to choose, our health care system will deteriorate to a level not seen in this century or the last.

I don't honestly think the public realizes that the rewards we seek as physicians are really not just financial. Yes, while we think we should be well compensated for years and years of personal sacrifice and training well into early middle age (my brother the heart surgeon, for instance, was making $22,000 twelve years after graduating from college), our true rewards come from the intimate involvement with the triumphs and tragedies in the lives of our patients. We became physicians because we realized that there are only a few ways, in the short span of time available to us, that we can truly touch the lives of those around us. And up to now, I have to say, it's been a ball!

But every doc I know is planning his alternative career, no kidding. My brother knows a forty-four-year-old general surgeon who just quit and opened a pizza parlor! I know of a plastic surgeon and his wife, an internist, who are planning to quit and teach high school. Another gynecologist at my hospital recently retired at forty-three and went into the computer software business. Another friend is considering quitting to raise cutting horses. Many are getting into multi-level marketing schemes. Some are branching out and trying to get into cash businesses like aesthetics including laser hair removal, dermabrasion and Botox. I even have a friend who left Ob/Gyn practice to go to law school and who is now . . . a plaintiff's attorney! For heaven's sake, some physicians even write books!

Lack of dedication, you say? I don't think so. Not after four years of college, four years of medical school, and three to seven years of residency. No, not lack of dedication, but lack of an attainable goal. The system is taking away the object of all those years of hard work. Managed competition will rob the physician of his most precious possession—his only true motivation. *It will rob him of his patient.*

Do not be confused by legislative debate on the national level. For the most part, it is the discussion of who will bear the brunt of the cost of expanding government's role in the delivery of health care. There are many published eloquent arguments debating universal coverage versus guaranteed coverage for single working moms and children, or the macroeconomic effect on our GNP of shifting an estimated $80 billion from upper income levels to lower, or the reasons behind the crumbling European socialized health care systems, or any of a myriad of other predominantly economic debates about how the haves will pay for the health of the have-nots.[39] But for the most part, the insidious process of converting American medicine from a physician-driven to a provider-driven system is occurring without government intervention. We are allowing it to occur by giving away our authority to make our own choices when we allow a corporate third party to foot the bill.

# Disrobe Completely

Oh, the medical profession will continue no matter what. Lawyers and insurance executives will continue to prosper from the new system. But if we're not careful, we won't have the best and the brightest at the other end of the stethoscope. We'll have a competent individual, happy to work from eight to five for the big company, caring not at all about patient rotation but valuing his job security and time off. In fact, we'll have just what the gentleman in the goatee at the managed care seminar suggested: a medical system whose physicians deliver a commodity just like every other businessman.

So get ready. It's coming. Unless you take action to stop it *proactively*, you're going to give up yet another freedom. You're going to give up the freedom to choose who touches you in the most private ways, who cares for you when you're miserable, who listens to you when you're down, who rejoices with you when you're well. And even worse, you're going to create a system in which you may be lucky to find in a physician the virtues that once were requisite.

An increasing number of patients across the United States, when faced with expensive surgeries for which coverage has been denied by their managed care provider, are seeking care overseas. Planethospital.com, for example, has been operating since 2002, arranging surgeries and medical therapies for Americans who can't afford to have the procedures they desperately need within our own system. Companies who promote "medical tourism" such as planethospital.com often escort their patients halfway around the world and provide excellent accommodations in modern hospital facilities with guaranteed follow-up afterwards for less than a third of what the cost would have been down the block from their homes. If ever there were a wake-up call to American legislators, this is one! Before long, the United States may no longer be the destination for sophisticated care but instead India, Belgium, Mexico, Singapore, Brazil, Uruguay, Argentina, etc. With over 45 million uninsured and many millions more who are insured but whose health plans decline to cover their need for a myriad of reasons, it is time to institute the kind of reforms we have discussed. From catastrophic poli-

# The Solution: Managed Competition?

cies with government-regulated premiums tied to inexpensive high-deductible HSAs to alterations of eligibility for and management of Medicaid dollars to changes in Medicare eligibility and patterns of compensation to elimination of pre-existing conditions to national tort reform, much needs to be done and done quickly!

# Conclusion

What can you do to preserve the finest health care system in the world? What can you do to keep compassion alive in the doctor-patient relationship? First, here's what you don't have to do.

You don't have to understand the intricacies of the on-again, off-again debates which rage in Washington, for even many of those embroiled in them do not.

You don't have to understand the intricacies of the myriad different managed competition paradigms proposed, as well as those already in existence.

You don't have to formulate your own plan for controlling health care costs while expanding care for the needy.

*The only thing you have to do is reject any scenario that restricts your choice of physician or facility.*

If one of your insurance choices includes such restrictions, I can assure you that the participating physicians have substantially lost their decision-making authority. Your health care will then be controlled by a corporate entity whose sole motivation is to be profitable.

Insist that your employer research and offer plans which do not restrict choice, even if those plans require large deductibles or involve employers contracting directly with health care systems. At the very least, the doctors from whom you currently receive care should be "grandfathered" for you in such a restrictive system. A choice with a large deductible may not seem financially possible on your income, but we know statistically that paying for your own routine health care out of pocket or out of money pooled and withheld by your employer must be cost effective, because the alternative, which includes filing a claim on relatively small outlays, generates huge profits for the insurers.

If you are self-employed or employed by a corporation who offers them, look seriously at phasing into an HSA for you and your family. You will quickly become a better health care consumer and save money for yourself and your employer while still maintaining your choice of physician and facility. If you find them unaffordable because of premium gouging for high-deductible insurance component, at least raise hell with your congressman and senator. Let them know that the insurer is working to disrupt a responsible linkage between true health care costs and your pocketbook! Let them know if your insurer doesn't allow HSA dollars spent to be applied to the deductible unless the provider is in the medical plan's network. Having a separate "out-of-net-work deductible" attached to HSA dollars is simply another way to subtly restrict choice and increase insurer's profits. If your employer offers an HSA option but does nothing to help you fund it, be as vocal as you can to management about your belief that helping all the employees to manage their own health care dollar would in very short order make up for the needed corporate contribution at the outset.

If you have no insurance, shop around for doctors and hospitals who charge much less if they simply know you are in a tight spot and need to pay cash. Despite ridiculous Medicare regulations that make it technically illegal for a doctor to have two fee scales (re discount anyone) almost all doctors and hospitals ignore this when it comes to cash discounts for the uninsured! Remember, doctor's fees are *artificially high* just as hospitals' fees are. Hospitals do so for cost shifting as previously explained, doctors do so because their negotiated rates for any service are downgraded by insurer's to some small percentage of their stated fees. For example, I might charge $2500 for a hysterectomy so that the negotiated managed care compensation is around $600. If you are paying cash, many ethical physicians would then only charge you the $600 they would have gotten from the insurer! Get it?

# Disrobe Completely

*Women, don't allow yourself to be forced into a situation where you do not have direct access to your Ob/Gyn.* You may have looked years before finding the doctor with whom you are really comfortable. As mentioned previously, 90% of your health problems under age fifty will fall within the expertise of your Ob/Gyn. There is no reason to accept an insurance plan of any sort that forces you to see a physician other than your Ob/Gyn for your routine care or gynecologic problems.

Managed care in some form is probably here to stay. If it is truly your only financially possible option, then look for systems with no "gatekeeper" component. Large, multi-specialty, physician-run HMOs *not* built on a "gate-keeper" model are more likely to deliver quality care, even if fully capitated, by avoiding the scenario where a screening physician decides if and/or which specialist you are permitted to see.

I urge women to write to their state legislators and support legislation that would mandate insurers granting unrestricted access to their Ob/Gyns at least once per year. California, Delaware, Georgia, Maryland, New York, Texas, and Virginia are among the first states to have passed some such legislation.

Our legislators should concentrate their efforts on plans which address only the indigent and working uninsured. Leave the rest of the system alone. They should give whatever incentives possible to small businesses who self-insure. Pooled withholdings to pay for outlays which fall into the deductible range of inexpensive catastrophic policies should be tax-free to the individual.

*Our nationwide county hospital/clinic system should be actively underwritten by the federal government.* It is a mistake to cripple these academic institutions by placing them in direct unrestricted competition with private hospitals involved in managed care contracting. It not only endangers excellent care now available to indigents, it directly threatens the survival of our country's university hospitals and graduate medical education programs. Neighborhood clinics involved in preventive health care should be expanded in all our metropolitan

# Conclusion

area, and ties to their associated university system strengthened.

Reform and/or federal regulation of the insurance industry is far beyond the scope of this text. However, *legislators should meet tomorrow and mandate the removal of all preexisting condition exclusions.* These are cruel. These are wrong. The burden could be equitably distributed to all of the companies in the industry. HIPAA did not come close to ending this problem.

Furthermore, policies should be truly portable. A job change should not affect an individual's health coverage unless the new job involves handling Uranium 238, waving red towels in front of angry bulls, or running tests on the Ebola virus. We could restore a little compassion right there. The Health-insurance Portability and Accountability Act (HIPAA) enacted on August 21, 1996, was intended to do just that. Unfortunately, Public Law 104–191, even after revisions in 2002, has become a giant, intrusive government behemoth. Strict enforcement of regulations regarding "privacy" have been taken to absurd extremes. My patients are well aware of the fact that they can't "sign in" at the front desk anymore because someone might "see" their name on the list and thus endanger their privacy; they are well aware that some hidden alarm will sound followed by public humiliation if they should inadvertently cross that red line on the floor ten feet back from the pharmacist's checkout counter while someone else is picking up a prescription! Unfortunately, they are also well aware that their insurance is NOT portable; that riders are placed on entire portions of their body for any history of preexisting problem, no matter how minor and no matter how absurd; and that changing jobs almost always involves changing insurers with exclusions to portions of their coverage. It seems that the "accountability" part is in full swing, but the "portability" part is nearly invisible.

# Disrobe Completely

Here's what you can do:

1. Actively oppose any proposal that limits your choices.

2. Actively pursue national tort reform.

3. Actively pursue means to re-connect *actual* health care costs to the consumer, such as *affordable* HRAs. This will move the nation away from its slide toward a one party, third party payor,(ie the federal government) toward a 300 million party payor where it should be! It will reinstate the authority for choice and payment to the patient where it belongs and remove it from the insurer.

4. Actively pursue private charitable means to help improve affordable access to health care for everyone.

5. Actively support legislative changes to eligibility for Medicare and Social Security which reflect increased years of working lives, and existing retirement income.

6. Encourage your legislature to *increase* Medicaid income eligibility limit of $20,000 to at least $30,000 for a family of four and put in place a system to review it periodically.

7. If you ARE currently uninsured, SHOP! Seek out cash discounts by comparing rates of doctors and hospitals who give substantial discounts to the uninsured. There really ARE compassionate people out there, you simply have to ASK!

8. Finally, support any measure to remove "health benefits" from corporate responsibility. Health benefits are killing American corporations. The responsibility should be on the individual to BUDGET for routine health costs and insure ONLY for catastrophe!

# Conclusion

## Final Thoughts

The world community still views health care in the United States as the best available anywhere, although many studies are beginning to challenge that due to our unequal access, poor infant mortality, huge per capita price, etc. But I firmly believe the success of our system thus far is rooted in the doctor-patient relationship. It is the joy of the art of healing that drives great minds, great medical education, and great research. If we destroy the joy of medicine for the physician, take away his relationship to the patient, and relegate him to the same position in the national psyche as any other worker, we will lose more than we ever thought possible.

In this great country, freedom of choice, whether related to speech, religion, education, or health care, is the foundation of our success. *Any proposals that significantly restrict your freedom to choose must be vigorously opposed.* The ideas put forth which limit your choice are the same ones which undermine the decision-making authority of our society's trained health professionals.

We must let neither the government nor our insurance companies undermine our liberty. In 1928, Justice Louis Brandeis said, "Experience should teach us to be most on our guard to protect our liberty when the government's [or insurance companies'] purposes are beneficent. The greatest dangers to liberty lurk in the insidious encroachment by men of zeal, well meaning, but without understanding."[40]

# Notes

1.  American College of Obstetricians & Gynecologists (ACOG) Technical Bulletins 1995.

2.  Maria Kassberg. "Turf War," *ObG Management* (October 1994) 46.

3.  Ibid.

4.  "NCI Changes Its Stance." *The Journal of the American Medical Association.* (12 January 1994) 271, 2: 96.

5.  A.B. Miller et al. "Canadian National Breast Cancer Screening Study." *Canadian Medical Association Journal.* (1992) 147: 1459–1476.

6.  K. Kerlilowsky, et al. "Positive Predictive Value of Screening Mammography by Age." *The Journal of the American Medical Association.* (1993) 270: 2444–2450.

7.  U. Smigel et al. "Canadian Mammogram Study to be Reviewed," *Journal of the National Cancer Institute.* (March 1995) 87, 6: 413.

8.  S. Shapiro. "Efficacy of Screening Mammography" and "Discussion." *Journal of the National Cancer Institute.* (November 1994) 86, 22: 1722–25.

9.  D.S. Greenberg. "NCI Blasted for Mammography Confusion." *Lancet.* (November 1994) 344, 8933: 1353.

10. J. Osuch et al. "Mammography Guidelines." *Cancer Journal for Clinicians.* (1994) 44, 5: 319.

11. Steve Parker. "Digital Stereotactic and Whole Breast Mammography." Lecture. February 3, 1995. Presbyterian Hospital, Dallas, Tex.

12. E.A. Sickles. "Mammographic Screening." *Annals of Internal Medicine.* (1 April 1995) 122, 7: 534–8.

13. V.G. Vogel. "Monographs." *National Cancer Institute.* (1994) 16: 55–60.

14. J. Kassirer. "Academic Medicine Under Siege." *The New England Journal of Medicine.* 1994. 331: 1370–1371.

14a. Weatherly, Leslie A., SPHR. "The rising cost of health care: strategic and societal considerations for employers." (August 2004) www.shrm.org/research/quarterly/q304health_essay.asp. pp. 1,5.

14b. "The U.S. Health-care System: Best in the World, or Just the Most Expensive?" Bureau of Labor Education, University of Maine. Public Service Document. (2001) 2.

15. "A Financial Overview of the Managed Care Industry." Fact Sheet, Kaiser Family Foundation. (March 1999). Information provided by Health-care Marketplace Project, Publication Number 1470.

16. Gerard F. Anderson, Peter S. Hussey, et al. "Health Spending in the United States and the Rest of the World." *Health Affairs.* 24, 4: 903–914.

17. Op. cit., Fact Sheet Kaiser Family Foundation.

18. Ibid, 3.

18a. George Anders. "As Patients, Doctors Feel Pinch, Insurer's CEO Makes a Billion." *Wall Street Journal.* (April 18, 2006) 1.

19. United States Congressional Report, sec. 6, "National Health-care and Medicare Spending." (June 2004) http://www.medpac.gov/publication/congressional_reports/Jun04DataBookSec6.pdf

20. Ibid, 2.

21. Health Systems Change News Release. "Physicians Still Welcome Medicare Patients." (January 9, 2006) http://www.hschange.org

# Notes

22. Luu, Than N. "Reducing the Costs of Civil Litigation." PLRI Public Law Research Institute, UC Hastings College of Law, San Francisco. (1995) http://w3.uchastings.edu/plri/fal95tex/cstslit.html

23. Conover, Christopher J. "Medical Tort System: Health Facilities Regulation Working Papers." No. MTS-1, Center for Health Policy, Law and Management, Duke University. (May 2004) 7.

24. American Medical Association. "America's Medical Liability Crisis." (February 2005) http://www.ama-assn.org/go/mlrnow.

25. Ibid., 2.

26. Andersen, Richard E. "Billions for Defense: The Pervasive Nature of Defensive Medicine." *Archives of Internal Medicine.* (8 November 1999) 159: 2399–2402.

27. Op cit. AMA, 2.

28. Leigh Page, *AMA News*, Oct 10, 1994.

29. Jones, Del. "Election Gives Hospital Giant More Clout." *USA Today,* (November 11, 1994) Sec. B.

30. Ibid.

31. Slomski, Anita. "How Business is Flattening Health Costs," *Medical Economics,* (August 1994) 2.

32. Ibid., 5.

32a. Op cit. Weatherly, 3

33. Ibid., 6.

34. Swartz, Mimi. "Not What the Doctor Ordered," *Texas Monthly* (March 1995) 116.

35.  Ibid., 115.

36.  "Eight Advantages of MSAs." *Physicians for Patient Power Newsletter.* (September 1994)

37.  Op cit., American Medical Association. pp. 2.

38.  Andersen. "Billions for Defense." 1.

39.  Reinhardt. "Coverage and Access in Health-care Reform." *The New England Journal of Medicine.* (May 19, 1994) 330, 20: 1452.

40.  Mark Head. Quoted in "The Two Minute Drill for Health Reform." (August 11, 1994)